THE CLINICAL LABORATORY MANUAL SERIES:

PHLEBOTOMY

D1716105

THE CLINICAL LABORATORY MANUAL SERIES:

PHLEBOTOMY

LYNN B. HOELTKE, M.B.A., M.T.(A.S.C.P.), P.B.T., D.L.M.

Delmar Publishers Inc.™

I(T)P™

NOTICE TO THE READER

Cover credit: Michael Traylor

Publishing Team:
Sponsoring Editor: Marion Waldman
Developmental Editor: Helen V. Yackel
Project Editor: Megan A. Terry
Production Coordinator: Jennifer L. Gaines
Art and Design Coordinator: Michael Traylor

Production Services: York Production Services

For information, address Delmar Publishers Inc.
3 Columbia Circle
Box 15015
Albany, NY 12212-5015

Printed in the United States of America
Published simultaneously in Canada
by Nelson Canada,
a division of the Thomson Corporation

1 2 3 4 5 6 7 8 9 10   XXX   01 00 99 98 97 96 95

Library of Congress Cataloging-in-Publication Data

Hoeltke, Lynn B.
    Clinical laboratory manual series : phlebotomy / by Lynn B. Hoeltke.
        p.   cm. — (Clinical laboratory manual series)
    Includes bibliographical references and index.
    ISBN 0-8273-5527-0
    1. Phlebotomy—Handbooks, manuals, etc.   I. Title.   II. Title: Phlebotomy.   III. Series.
    [DNLM: 1. Bloodletting—examination questions.   WB 18 H694c 1995]
    RB45.15.H64   1995
    616.07'561—dc20
    DNLM/DLC
    for Library of Congress   93-46473
                                                               CIP

Other Delmar titles in this Clinical Laboratory Manual Series include:

Marshall/The Clinical Laboratory Manual Series: Microbiology
Smith/The Clinical Laboratory Manual Series: Immunology

Also available from Delmar Publishers:

Marshall/Fundamental Skills for the Clinical Laboratory Professional
Hoeltke/The Complete Textbook of Phlebotomy
Fong/Lakomia/Microbiology for Health Careers, 5E
Walters/Basic Medical Laboratory Techniques, 2E

TABLE OF CONTENTS

PREFACE

The *Clinical Laboratory Manual Series* is designed for use by instructors in vocational schools, community colleges, and the clinical laboratory environment to give the medical laboratory technician the best training possible to keep up with the demands of the rapidly changing health care environment. Safety issues are strongly emphasized in all manuals.

The *Phlebotomy Manual* of this series strongly emphasizes a hands-on practical approach to learning. Manual exercises are woven throughout the instructional materials to enhance this learning. Traditionally, the task of phlebotomy was centralized in the clinical laboratory, with training done informally, on the job, in a sink-or-swim manner. The task of phlebotomy is now decentralized and performed by many types of crosstrained individuals, from nurses on hospital wards to associates working in outpatient settings.

In writing this book, standards have been used to establish criteria for the proper collection of blood specimens. The National Committee for Clinical Laboratory Standards (NCCLS) and the Federal Register detailing Occupational Safety and Health Administration (OSHA) rules and regulations are used as the primary references for establishing proper procedures. Health care centers follow these standards and regulations. By following them and by knowing the importance of proper specimen collection we can provide patients with the highest quality of care available. Developing the phlebotomist's ability to improve patient care is the main purpose of this book.

The manual is divided into six Units: Introduction to Phlebotomy, Safety in Phlebotomy, Phlebotomy Equipment, Phlebotomy Technique, The Challenging Phlebotomy, and Specimen Considerations and Special Procedures. Each Unit contains Learning Objectives, a Glossary, Exercises, Review Questions, and Further Activities.

Lynn B. Hoeltke

The following reviewers contributed significantly to the development of this manual:

Professor John O'Leary
Hudson Valley Community College
Albany, NY

Margaret Tarr (Retired)
Floyd Knobs, IN

Patrick Shen PhD
Department of Medical Laboratory Sciences
Florida International University
Miami, FL

JoAnne Rademaker M.T. ASCP
Northwest Hospital
Seattle, WA

Lisa Shimeld
Department Head, Biological Sciences
Crafton Hills College
Yucaipa, CA

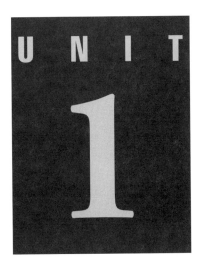

UNIT 1

Introduction to Phlebotomy

LEARNING OBJECTIVES

After studying this unit, it is the responsibility of the student to know the following objectives:

- Identify the reason blood is collected by the phlebotomist today.

- Explain the responsibility of the phlebotomist to the patient with regard to the reliability of the phlebotomist's work and respect of the patient as a human being.

- Explain why the phlebotomist has a special responsibility to present a neat, pleasant, and competent demeanor.

- Identify departments within the hospital and explain their function.

- Identify each section of the laboratory.

- Define ethics.

- List five patient rights.

- Describe the characteristics of the different types of blood cells.

- Differentiate between serum and plasma.

GLOSSARY

Erythrocytes	Also known as red blood cells.
Ethics	Professional code of conduct in treatment of patients.

Leukocytes	Also known as white blood cells
Phlebotomy	Act or practice of bloodletting as a therapeutic measure.
Thrombocytes	Also known as platelets.

INTRODUCTION

The laboratory professional who performs the task of collecting blood samples from patients is the phlebotomist. The phlebotomist is an important part of the health care team. Without the blood samples obtained by the phlebotomist, the physician would have few means to diagnose a patient's disease.

The phlebotomist is the laboratory representative. Often the phlebotomist is the only laboratory associate that has contact with the patient.

WHY COLLECT BLOOD?

Phlebotomy, the process of collecting blood, is defined by Webster's dictionary as "the act or practice of bloodletting as a therapeutic measure." The history of bloodletting dates back to the early Egyptians, and the practice continues into modern times. Phlebotomy in the past was the method to cure individuals. Phlebotomy is now used to determine the disease process taking place and is used to determine the method of cure.

PHLEBOTOMY'S ROLE IN HEALTH CARE

The phlebotomist's primary role is to collect blood for accurate and reliable test results as quickly as possible. The job can vary greatly from one health care environment to another. Phlebotomists represent the laboratory and the health care center, they directly contact the patient, and they perform tasks that are critical to the patient's diagnosis and care. Phlebotomists are a part of a health care team that can be as large as 5,000 people in a large hospital, or 2 or 3 in a small clinic. The larger the institution, the more complex the organization.

A laboratory organization forms a pyramid, with the number of individuals increasing as you move toward the base of the pyramid. The laboratory organizational chart usually contains a smaller side pyramid that includes the pathologists and their relationship to the rest of the laboratory staff. This relationship is shown as a dotted line. Figure 1.1 shows a typical organizational chart.

The laboratory has to have organization for the team of laboratory professionals to function smoothly. The interaction has developed into an organizational chart for the laboratory. The organization of the laboratory delineates the tasks to be performed, the individuals who are to perform the tasks, and the clinical laboratory as a workplace.

The clinical laboratory can be in one location or decentralized into the main laboratory, ambulatory care laboratory (outpatient laboratory), a stat laboratory or the surgery laboratory. Each laboratory serves a specific function and often has sections within it (Table 1.1).

E X E R C I S E ORGANIZATIONAL CHART

Talk to the director of a local laboratory to learn how many levels are in that laboratory's organization.

E X E R C I S E **2** HOSPITAL DEPARTMENTS

Divide the class into four groups. Each group reports back to the class:

1. A hospital department other than nursing service they would relate to as a phlebotomist.
2. What working relationship they would have with this department.

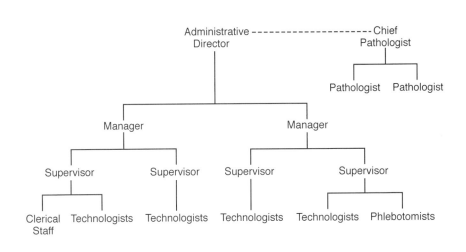

fig **1.1** Laboratory organizational chart

Even with the elaborate testing facilities available in most laboratories, outside laboratories are often needed to do specialized testing. These reference laboratories can be in the same city or many miles away. The specimens are transported to the reference laboratory each evening, and results are sent back by way of computer and telephone lines the next morning.

The phlebotomy section is the one emphasized in this manual. The goal of the phlebotomist is to provide specimens for accurate and reliable test results as quickly as possible.

EXERCISE **3** ## HOSPITAL NURSING

Have a nurse from a local hospital tell about nursing and how the nurse relates to the phlebotomist.

EXERCISE **4** ## CLINICAL LABORATORY

Tour a local hospital. Include the laboratory and different hospital departments.

Table 1–1 Sections Within a Laboratory

1. Blood bank (immunohematology)
2. Chemistry
3. Coagulation
4. Hematology
5. Immunology
6. Microbiology
7. Phlebotomy
8. Urinalysis

The requirements to be a phlebotomist include:

1 High school education
2 Specialized training in phlebotomy consisting of a minimum of:
  a. 40 hours of classroom training
  b. 120 hours of clinical or practical training

Many hospitals have established training programs to fill phlebotomy positions. Phlebotomists are now taking certification exams to prove their knowledge in phlebotomy. A variety of certification and registry exams can be taken to classify a person as a phlebotomy technician. See Appendix A.

EXERCISE **PHLEBOTOMIST**

1. Call a local hospital personnel department and ask for a phlebotomist job description.
2. Compare the duties listed in job descriptions from different hospitals.

EXERCISE **PHLEBOTOMIST CERTIFICATION**

Divide the class into groups. Each group inquires with a different phlebotomy certification agency for the requirements for certification.

ETHICAL CONSIDERATIONS

The phlebotomist is intricately involved with ethics and sees ethical decisions being made daily. **Ethics** consists of more than a set of written rules, procedures, or guidelines. Ingrained in ethics is a moral philosophy that varies by individual, religion, social status, or heritage. Ethics requires that the phlebotomist act responsibly to the patient to provide high-quality patient care. Acting ethically is a standard of conduct a phlebotomist must follow when working with patients and the public. Following this code of ethics is being professional.

Daily patient contact makes the phlebotomist unique among the laboratory associates. Phlebotomists have to put up with the worst in human behavior. Many patients do not want the phlebotomist to even come near them, and often phlebotomists have to talk patients into letting them draw the blood. The nicest patient will often be irritable and may even physically and emotionally abuse the phlebotomist when placed in the strange world of the hospital. With this type of abuse, the phlebotomist may find it difficult to be ethical and professional with the patient. The phlebotomist must remember the patient is the customer and has patient rights. See Appendix B.

The patient is often apprehensive about the procedure being performed. It is important not only to obtain a good specimen but also to do so with minimal trauma to the patient. The patient must be treated as anyone would like to be treated. This is the key to ethical treatment of patients.

STANDARDS USED IN THE LABORATORY

A large body of regulations governs laboratories, and a variety of agencies issue these regulations and standards (Table 1.2). A laboratory accepting Medicare or Medicaid reim-

EXERCISE 7 PATIENT RIGHTS

Divide the class into pairs. Each pair role plays, with one student being the patient and the other student the phlebotomist. Each pair will have a discussion of the patient asking the phlebotomist about one of the patient rights.

EXERCISE 8 ETHICS

Divide the class into three teams. Each team discusses an ethical situation and reports back to the class.

1. How can a phlebotomist be professional to a rude patient?
2. What should the phlebotomist do if a friend from outside of the hospital asks the phlebotomist to find out confidential information about a patient in the hospital?
3. There is a celebrity in the hospital. A reporter stops the phlebotomist leaving the hospital and asks questions about the celebrity.

bursement must meet all applicable state and local requirements and must be accredited by the appropriate agency.

BODY SYSTEMS

The human body has a variety of body systems (Table 1.3). The body maintains an internal environment consisting of many processes that work both independently and together to maintain an equilibrium. The phlebotomist collects blood samples whose results indicate to the physician how different body systems are out of balance.

ANATOMY AND PHYSIOLOGY OF THE CIRCULATORY SYSTEM

To be prepared to collect blood, the phlebotomist must understand the system that carries this blood. This system is the circulatory system. Blood forms in the organs of the body. The bone marrow is the primary factory for production of blood cells. The lymph nodes, thymus, and spleen are also sites for the production of white blood cells. The function of

Table `1-2` Agencies That Set Standards for Health Care

1. Joint Commission on Accreditation of Health Care Organizations (JCAHO)
2. American Osteopathic Association (AOA)
3. College of American Pathologists (CAP)
4. State Board of Health
5. National Committee for Clinical Laboratory Standards (NCCLS)
6. Clinical Laboratory Improvement Act (CLIA) of 1967
7. Clinical Laboratory Improvement Act of 1988
8. Occupational Safety and Health Act (OSHA)

Table `1-3` Body Systems

1. Skeletal
2. Muscular
3. Nervous
4. Respiratory
5. Urinary
6. Digestive
7. Endocrine
8. Reproductive
9. Circulatory

Erythrocytes
(Red Blood Cells)

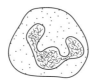

Leukocytes
(White Blood Cells)

Thrombocytes
(Platelets)

fig `1.2` Formed cellular elements in peripheral blood

the red blood cells is to carry oxygen to body tissues and to remove the waste product, carbon dioxide. The blood also carries nutrients to all parts of the body and moves the waste products to the lungs, kidneys, liver, and skin to eliminate them. The main function of the circulatory system is to provide transportation.

The body contains approximately 6 liters of blood, 45 percent of which consists of formed elements. The formed cellular elements are **erythrocytes** (red blood cells), **leukocytes** (white blood cells), and **thrombocytes** (platelets), (Figs. 1.2 and 1.3; Table 1.4).

The heart pumps the blood through the body by way of tubing called arteries, veins, and

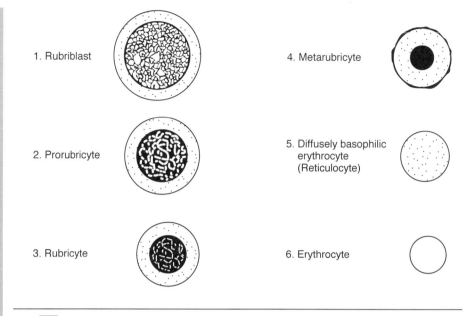

1. Rubriblast

2. Prorubricyte

3. Rubricyte

4. Metarubricyte

5. Diffusely basophilic erythrocyte (Reticulocyte)

6. Erythrocyte

fig `1.3` Erythrocyte maturation

Table `1–4` Cellular Elements of the Blood

	Leukocytes (White Blood Cells)	**Erythrocytes (Red Blood Cells)**	**Thrombocytes (Platelets)**
Function	Body defense (extravascular) (intravascular)	Transport of oxygen and carbon dioxide	Stoppage of bleeding
Formation	Bone marrow, lymphatic tissue	Bone marrow	Bone marrow
Size/shape	9–16 micrometers; different size, shape, color, nucleus (core) in blood	6–7 micrometers; biconcave disc. Normally no nucleus	1–4 micrometers; fragments of megakaryocytes
Life cycle	Varies, 24 hours–years	100–120 days	9–12 days
Numbers	5–10,000 per cubic millimeter	4.5–5.5 million per cubic millimeter	250–450,000 per cubic millimeter
Removal	Bone marrow, liver, spleen	Bone marrow, spleen	Spleen

capillaries. Blood flowing away from the heart flows in the arteries. Blood flowing back to the heart flows in the veins. Connecting most of the arteries and veins are the capillaries (Fig. 1.4 and Table 1.5).

The artery has a thick wall that helps it withstand the pressure of the pumping of the heart. The arteries branch to form arterioles, which branch more to become capillaries. The capillaries then start converging to form venules, and the venules then become veins. As blood flows through the body it follows this path of artery–capillary–vein. Oxygenated arterial blood leaves the heart and carries this oxygen to the tissue by releasing the oxygen

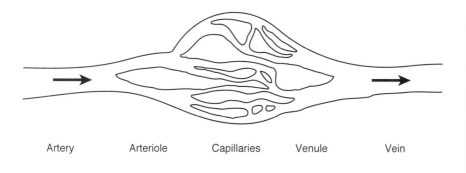

Artery　　Arteriole　　Capillaries　　Venule　　Vein

fig 1.4 Blood flow

Table 1–5 Arteries versus Veins

Arteries	Veins
1. Carry blood from the heart, carry oxygenated blood (except pulmonary artery)	1. Carry blood to the heart, carry deoxygenated blood (except pulmonary vein)
2. Normally bright red in color	2. Normally dark red in color
3. Elastic walls that expand with surge of blood	3. Thin walls/less elastic
4. No valves	4. Valves
5. Can feel a pulse	5. No pulse

through the cell walls of the capillaries. At the same time, carbon dioxide is being absorbed by the blood and then transported to the lungs to be exhaled as a waste product. The flow of the blood also regulates body temperature. When the body gets warm the capillaries in the extremities dilate (enlarge in diameter) and let off heat. This process then cools the body. If the body becomes cold, the capillaries constrict (get smaller in diameter), and less blood will flow through, therefore conserving heat for the rest of the body.

The formed elements of the blood make up only 45 percent of the total volume. The remaining 55 percent is liquid. Generally, 2 milliliters of blood will yield about 1 milliliter of fluid. In the body, the liquid portion is called plasma. When the blood is removed from the body, the blood clots and the liquid portion is called serum. The clot contains all the formed elements intertwined in a fibrin mass. Blood that is flowing through the body contains a substance called fibrinogen. Once the blood leaves the body, the fibrinogen turns into fibrin. This fibrin is like a sticky spider web and traps the formed elements into the fibrin mass called a clot. The clot then will contract and the liquid (serum) portion can be extracted. This serum is a clear straw-colored liquid that is used for many of the tests done in the laboratory. To speed removal of the serum, an instrument called a centrifuge spins the blood. A carrier holds the tubes of blood; when the centrifuge is started, the carrier spins. The spinning carrier pushes the blood to the bottom of the tube. The blood separates according to weight. The clot will go to the bottom of the tube, and the serum will be on the top layer.

EXERCISE **9** VIEWING FORMED ELEMENTS WITH THE COMPOUND MICROSCOPE

Examine a blood smear with a microscope.

1. With clean hands, make sure the oculars and objectives are clean. Clean them with lens paper.

2. Using the coarse adjustment, raise the nosepiece unit. Raise the condenser as far as possible by turning the condenser knob.

3. Rotate the low-power objective (10×) into position so it is directly over the opening in the stage, turn on the microscope light.

4. Open the diaphragm until maximum light comes through the condenser.

5. Put the stained blood smear provided by your instructor on the microscope stage and secure with clips. The condenser should be in a position to almost touch the slide bottom.

6. Find the coarse adjustment. Looking at the stage and the low-power objective (10×), turn the coarse adjustment until the objective is as close to the stage as possible.

7. Look into the oculars (you may have to adjust the distance between oculars for your eyes so that only one image is seen) and slowly turn the adjustment in the opposite direction to raise the objective until the blood cells come into focus.

8. Locate the fine adjustment. Use both coarse and and fine adjustments to bring the blood cells into correct focus while looking through the right ocular with only the right eye.

9. Close the right eye and look into the left ocular with the left eye. Use the collar on the left ocular to bring the blood cells into sharp focus, not using the coarse or fine adjustments. Now check to see with both eyes that the objects are in clear focus.

10. Using the stage control knobs, scan the slide by moving the slide left and right and backward and forward while looking through the oculars.

11. Rotate the high-power objective (40×) into place while observing the objective and the slide to ensure the objective does not hit the slide.

12. Look through the oculars to view the blood cells on the slide, which should be almost in focus. Focus further with the fine adjustment. Do *not* use the coarse adjustment.

<table>
<tr><td>E X E R C I S E</td><td>9</td><td>VIEWING FORMED ELEMENTS WITH
THE COMPOUND MICROSCOPE
(CONT'D)</td></tr>
</table>

13. Scan the slide. Rotate the oil immersion ($100\times$) objective to the side so that no objective is in position. Place a drop of immersion oil on the portion of the slide directly over the condenser.

14. Rotate the oil immersion objective into position, being careful not to move the $40\times$ objective through the oil. Observe to see that the oil immersion objective is touching the oil drop.

15. Look through the oculars and slowly turn the fine adjustment until the blood cells are in focus. Do not use the coarse adjustment.

16. Scan the slide to see the different types of leukocytes.

17. After viewing, rotate the $10\times$ objective into position, not allowing the $40\times$ objective to pass through the oil.

18. Remove the slide from the stage and gently clean the oculars, wiping any oil from the slide, stage, and condenser with lens paper.

19. Turn off the microscope light and disconnect the microscope, making sure the nosepiece is positioned in the lowest position using the coarse adjustment.

20. Center the stage so there is no projection from either side, and cover the microscope if it will not be used for several hours.

21. In your notebook, make a drawing of what you saw in this exercise.

To produce a plasma specimen, the blood has to be prevented from clotting. An anticoagulant is a chemical substance that prevents the blood from clotting. An anticoagulated tube of blood that has been centrifuged will layer the formed elements and plasma according to weight. The bottom layer will contain the erythrocytes; then there will be a thin layer called the buffy coat. The buffy coat contains a mixture of leukocytes and thrombocytes. On top of all these layers is the plasma layer. The plasma contains fibrinogen and usually is slightly hazy (Fig. 1.6).

The bend of the arm is the usual location that the phlebotomist chooses to draw blood. The veins are near the surface and large enough to give access to the blood (Fig. 1.7). The median cubital vein is the vein that is used the majority of the time. When this vein is not available, any of the other veins that can be felt may be used. These veins include the basilic, cephalic, median, and median cephalic. The superficial veins in the hand require special techniques for collection.

The arteries in the arm consist of the brachial artery in the brachial region of the arm and the radial and ulnar arteries in the wrist (Fig. 1.8). Puncturing of arteries require special techniques used when obtaining a blood gas specimen. Arterial punctures and the techniques used to draw blood from these locations for blood gas testing are explained in Unit 4.

UNIT 1 ■

EXERCISE 10 CENTRIFUGING

Centrifuge several different blood samples.

1. The principle of "balance" must be observed. Tubes and carriers of equal weight, size, and shape must be placed in opposing positions in the centrifuge head.
2. Select blood tubes provided by your instructor for centrifugation.
3. All blood tubes must be stoppered.
4. Pair the tubes by size, shape, and amount of blood. Tubes that match are placed in opposing positions in the carriers (Fig. 1.5). If there is a tube that does not have a match, fill an opposing tube with water to achieve a match.
5. The tube carriers are then covered to prevent aerosols if the carriers are equipped with covers.
6. The lid of the centrifuge is then closed and locked.
7. The desired time for centrifugation is then set on the centrifuge, or a separate timer is set.
8. The centrifuge is slowly accelerated until maximum desired speed is obtained.
9. The centrifuge will automatically turn off at the preset time, or if a separate timer is set, turn off the centrifuge after the desired time.
10. Do not slow the centrifuge with a brake; this will cause the centrifuged specimens to be resuspended.
11. Do not try to open the lid until the centrifuge has come to a complete stop.
12. Open the lid of the centrifuge and remove the carrier covers.
13. Lift the tubes out of the carriers.
14. Do not agitate the tubes or tilt the tubes on their sides.
15. Place the tubes in a test-tube rack for observation.
16. Examine the samples for the different layering and coloration of the layers.
17. In your notebook, make a drawing of what you saw in this exercise.

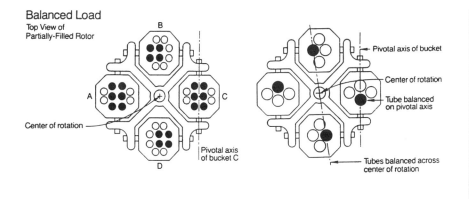

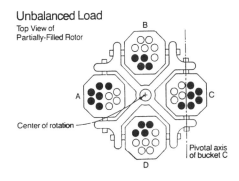

fig 1.5 Centrifuge balance

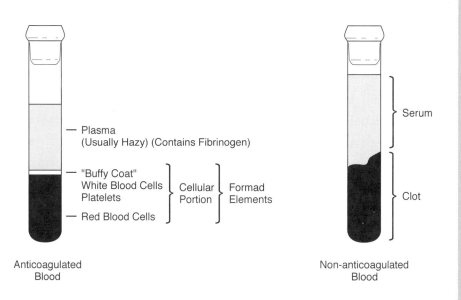

fig 1.6 Blood tubes

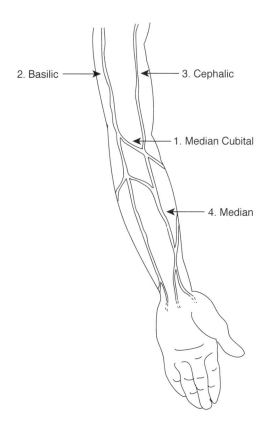

fig **1.7** Superficial veins of the arm and hand

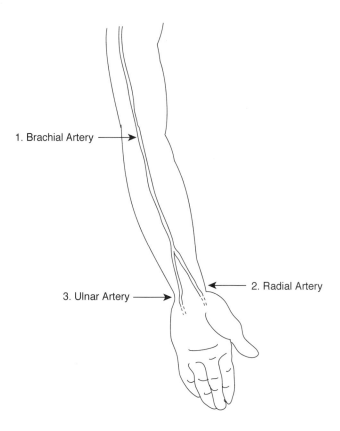

fig **1.8** Arteries of the arm

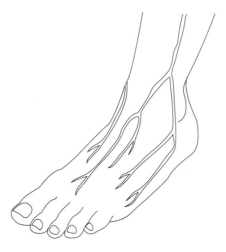

fig 1.9 Superficial veins of the legs and feet

The veins of the feet are an alternative when the arms are not available. A physician's permission is needed before drawing blood from the veins of the legs and feet (Fig. 1.9). The physician may not want the patient's leg or foot veins punctured because the act of drawing blood may cause clots to form. These clots then have the possibility of dislodging and causing a blockage elsewhere in the body.

SUMMARY

The phlebotomist's primary role is to collect blood for accurate and reliable test results as quickly as possible. Daily patient contact makes the phlebotomist unique among the laboratory associates. Phlebotomists have to put up with the worst in human behavior. Many patients do not want the phlebotomist even to come near them, and the phlebotomist often has to talk the patient into letting blood be drawn. The phlebotomist may find it difficult to be ethical and professional with the patient at all times. The phlebotomist must remember the patient is the customer and has patient rights.

The phlebotomist must know about the circulatory system of the body. The function of the circulatory system is to provide transportation for formed cellular elements. The process of drawing blood is an invasive procedure in which the phlebotomist accesses veins of this circulatory system to obtain a blood sample.

The body contains approximately 6 liters of blood, 45 percent of which consists of formed elements. The formed cellular elements are erythrocytes (red blood cells), leukocytes (white blood cells), and thrombocytes (platelets).

The blood specimens the phlebotomist obtains consist of anticoagulated or clotted blood specimens. The fluid portion of the anticoagulated blood specimen is plasma; the fluid from the clotted blood specimen is serum.

REVIEW QUESTIONS

Choose the one best answer.

1 The formed elements make up about _____ percent of the whole blood volume.
a. 30
b. 60
c. 55
d. 45

2 The two components of blood found in a tube of blood drawn *without* anticoagulant are
a. plasma and clot.
b. buffy coat and erythrocytes.
c. serum and buffy coat.
d. serum and clot.

3 The difference between plasma and serum is
a. serum comes from anticoagulated blood, and plasma does not.
b. plasma contains fibrinogen, and serum does not.
c. serum contains fibrinogen, and plasma does not.
d. plasma is found only inside the body.

4 The fluid portion of the whole blood that contains fibrinogen is called
a. buffy coat.
b. erythrocytes.
c. plasma.
d. serum.

5 The fluid portion of blood after clotting has taken place is called
a. buffy coat.
b. erythrocytes.
c. plasma.
d. serum.

6 The main function of the circulatory system is to provide
a. absorption.
b. elimination.
c. protection.
d. transportation.

FURTHER ACTIVITIES

Go to the library to locate information on CLIA 1988 and write a paper on how CLIA 1988 is affecting laboratories today.

Discuss each of the body systems and how each body system affects other body systems.

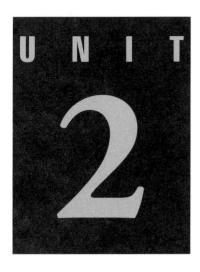

Safety in Phlebotomy

LEARNING OBJECTIVES

After studying this unit, it is the responsibility of the student to know the following objectives:

■ Identify rules of safety that promote safety of the individual and patient.

■ Explain the principle and procedures for infection control.

■ Describe the proper handwashing technique and when to use this technique.

■ Explain the concept of infection.

■ List the eight types of isolation.

■ Explain the purpose and scope of Universal Precautions.

■ Describe precautionary measures and actions to be taken with accidental needle punctures.

■ Explain the purpose of Material-Safety Data Sheets (MSDS).

GLOSSARY

Autoclave	A container for sterilizing using steam under pressure.
Biohazard	Anything that is potentially hazardous to humans, living organisms, or the environment.
Hazardous Chemical	Any element, chemical compound, or mixture of elements and/or compounds that causes physical or health hazards.

Nosocomial Infection	Infection as a result of a stay in a health care facility.
Sharps Container	Specially labeled puncture-resistant containers for the disposal of sharp items such as needles, scalpels, and syringes.

I N T R O D U C T I O N

Maintaining a safe working environment is of primary concern for all who work in or have exposure in the health care industry. Standards and procedures need to be formalized to protect the laboratory professional and the patient. These procedures are often established to protect the laboratory professional from being infected by the patient. The procedures also protect the patient from being infected by the laboratory professional or other patients.

INFECTION CONTROL AND ISOLATION TECHNIQUES

A patient that comes into a hospital and develops an infection as a result of the stay in the hospital is said to have obtained a **nosocomial infection**.

Handwashing

Handwashing is the single most important means of preventing the spread of infection. Hands must be washed after each patient contact, even when gloves are used. Hands must be washed under running water with soap and vigorous rubbing. When the soap is rinsed off, the water should flow from the wrists to the fingertips. Disinfectant waterless hand cleaners are used only when running water is not available.

Preventing the Spread of Infection

The spread of infection requires a source of infecting organisms, a susceptible host, and a means of transmission of the organism. Connecting these three factors are two different

E X E R C I S E 11 NOSOCOMIAL INFECTIONS

Divide the class into groups to discuss how the phlebotomist could cause a nosocomial infection with:

1. The phlebotomy tray
2. Tourniquet
3. Not changing gloves
4. Not washing hands

portals. There is a portal of exit from the source and a portal of entry into the susceptible host. This creates a chain:

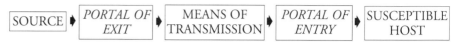

The source of an infection can be health care associates, other patients, or visitors. The source can have an active acute infection or be carrying the infection and not realize he or she has it. With the number of people contacting each other in a health care setting, the potential is great for the chain of infection to be started.

The means of transmission is where the health care team works to break the chain of infection. To do this, the patient is often placed in isolation (Table 2.1). Isolation limits the amount of contact time a patient has to spread an infection. This isolation can be used to prevent the patient from spreading an infection to associates, other patients, or visitors. Isolation can also be used to prevent the spread of an infection to the patient. Handwashings between patients and using a new pair of gloves with each patient are the most critical elements the phlebotomist can use to prevent the spread of infection.

EXERCISE 12 — HANDWASHING TECHNIQUE

1. Stand at sink and turn faucets on using paper toweling to avoid direct contact with the faucets. Adjust water temperature to moderately warm and discard paper towels.

2. Wet hands and press soap dispenser to obtain approximately 1 teaspoon of soap in the palm of one hand. Work soap into lather and distribute soap over both palms and backs of hands in circular motion constantly and vigorously for 2 minutes.

3. Rinse well, being careful not to touch inside of sink or faucets during procedure.

EXERCISE 13 — SOURCES OF INFECTION

Divide the class into groups. Each group demonstrates to the class:

1. A possible source of infection.

2. How to prevent the infection.

Table 2.1 gives a list of types of isolation. Many hospitals have simplified this list to include only strict isolation and reverse isolation.

Blood-borne pathogens such as hepatitis B virus (HBV) or human immunodeficiency virus (HIV) cannot always readily be detected. Therefore, a safety standard called *Universal Precautions* has been established by the Center for Disease Control (CDC). This standard states that all patients are considered potentially infectious for HBV or HIV and all body substances must be treated as infectious. It is recommended that Universal Precautions be used when working with any body fluid or unfixed tissue (Table 2.2).

Most health care organizations use a blend of Universal Precautions and specific disease-related isolation. Patients that have a known disease that is infectious are placed in the proper isolation. Several methods are used to tell the phlebotomist what type of isolation is present and what precautions should be taken before entering the room (Figs. 2.2 and 2.3). All other patients, whether in isolation or not, are treated according to Universal Precautions.

The rubber stopper on the tube has changed with the increase of blood and body-fluid precautions. The traditional rubber stopper would "pop" as the top was removed to access the specimen. This would create an aerosol that could be inhaled or ingested. The Becton

---

Table **2–1** Eight Types of Isolation

Type of isolation	Reason
Strict isolation	Highly contagious disease
Contact isolation	Scabies infection
Respiratory isolation	Mumps, pertussis, rubella
Tuberculosis isolation	Tuberculosis infection
Drainage/secretion precautions	Wound drainage
Enteric precautions	Fecal contamination
Protective or reverse isolation	Protecting the patient
Blood and body-fluid precautions	Body-fluid contamination

Table  **2–2** Universal Precaution Requirements

1 Wash hands when changing gloves and between patients.

2 Wear gloves when likely to touch body substances, mucous membranes, or nonintact skin and during all blood drawing.

3 Wear protective cover when clothing is likely to be soiled.

4 Wear mask/eye protection in addition to protective body cover when likely to be splashed with body substances.

5 Needles, scalpels, disposable syringes with needle still attached, and any other sharp items are placed in a puncture-resistant **sharps container** (Fig. 2.1). Do not bend, break, or cut needles.

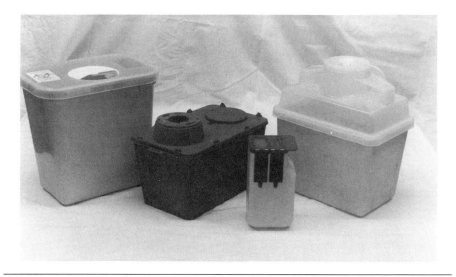

fig 2.1 Sharps container

Respiratory Isolation
Visitors—Report to Nurses' Station Before Entering Room

1. PRIVATE ROOM—Necessary; door must be kept closed
2. GOWNS—Not necessary
3. MASKS—Must be worn by all persons entering room if susceptible to disease
4. HANDS—Must be washed on entering and leaving room
5. GLOVES—Not necessary
6. ARTICLES—Those contaminated with secretions must be disinfected
7. CAUTION—All persons susceptible to the specific disease should be excluded from patient area; if contact is necessary, susceptibles must wear masks

---

fig 2.2 Respiratory isolation card

Dickinson Company developed a tube they named Hemogard (Fig. 2.4). This tube has a plastic sleeve that fits over the rubber stopper to contain any aerosols that might be dispersed when the cap is removed. Although the Hemogard cap does not make drawing blood easier, it is used for the safety of the person handling the sample.

Tubes made from plastic are now being used more frequently in health care locations that experienced an abnormal amount of tube breakage. Only recently have plastics been developed that can maintain a vacuum within the tube. Plastic tubes are manufactured with or without anticoagulant. Another innovation incorporated into some plastic tubes is a peel-off stopper. The peel-off stopper has a thinner rubber seal to make piercing the stopper while drawing blood easier (Fig. 2.5).

Drawing Blood From a Patient in Isolation

The collection of blood from a patient in an isolation room requires a specific procedure. This procedure is easiest when two people are available; one individual can receive the tubes of blood in a sealable plastic transport bag at the door. Used articles must be enclosed in an impervious bag before they are removed from the isolation room. This bagging pre-

Visitors—Report to Nurses' Station Before Entering Room

1. Private room indicated?   ____ No
     ____ Yes

2. Masks indicated?   ____ No
     ____ Yes for those close to patient
     ____ Yes for all persons entering room

3. Gowns indicated?   ____ No
     ____ Yes if soiling is likely
     ____ Yes for all persons entering room

4. Gloves indicated?   ____ No
     ____ Yes for touching infective material
     ____ Yes for all persons entering room

5. Special precautions indicated for handling blood?   ____ No
     ____ Yes

6. Hands must be washed after touching the patient or potentially contaminated articles and before taking care of another patient.

7. Articles contaminated with infective material(s) should be red-bagged and discarded or red-bagged and labeled before being sent for decontamination and reprocessing.

Instructions

1. On the table Disease-Specific Isolation Precautions, locate the disease for which isolation precautions are indicated.

2. Write disease in blank space here:

3. Determine if a private room is indicated. In general, patients infected with the same organism may share a room. For some diseases or conditions, a private room is indicated if patient hygiene is poor (infants, children, altered mental status, etc). A patient with poor hygiene does not wash hands after touching infective material (feces, purulent drainage, or secretions), contaminates the environment with infective material, or shares contaminated articles with other patients.

4. Place a check mark beside the indicated precautions on front of card.

5. Cross through precautions that are not indicated.

6. Write infective material in blank space in item 7 on front of card.

fig 2.3 Disease-specific isolation

vents exposure of associates to the contaminated materials. A double-bagging method is used. The articles bagged in the isolation room are sealed, and the bag is dropped into a bag held by an individual outside the room. The double-bagged articles can then be transported without the possibility of contamination. In reality, two associates are not usually available, and a modification of the double-bagging technique is necessary. The procedure in Exercise 15 has been developed for the phlebotomist working alone.

OCCUPATIONAL SAFETY AND HEALTH ADMINISTRATION (OSHA) STANDARDS

The Occupational Safety and Health Administration (OSHA) is an agency of the federal government that investigates the possibility of unsafe practices in the work environment. The OSHA regulations are for the protection of the health care worker. The rules and regulations that health care institutions must comply with are published in a government pub-

EXERCISE **14** PROTECTIVE CLOTHING FOR ISOLATION

1. Wash hands.

2. Remove lab coat.

3. Pick up protective gown, being careful it does not touch the floor. Hold the gown from the inside and place arms in sleeves. The opening of the gown must be in back.

4. Tie the neck ties and then the waist.

5. Pick up the mask by the ties. Hold it so the correct side is on the outside.

6. The mask is tied high on the head so it will not slip. Most masks have a metal band that fits over the nose. Bend this band for a snug fit over the nose.

7. Goggles or safety glasses must also be worn when there is a chance for spattering of body fluids. Place them over the eyes so that any spattering will not enter around the glasses. Some masks now are equipped with safety shields that cover and protect the eyes. These can be used instead of a mask and goggles.

8. Put on the gloves. Pull the cuff of the glove over the sleeve of the gown.

9. To remove the protective clothing, first untie the gown at the waist for gowns that tie in the front. If the gown ties in the back, remove gloves first.

10. Remove the gloves by slipping a finger under the cuff of one glove, pulling this glove off inside out. This glove is then held in a ball in the gloved hand. With the ungloved hand, place a finger under the cuff of the remaining glove, pulling this glove off inside out. The first glove removed should now be bagged in the second glove. Deposit in appropriate waste receptacle.

11. Remove goggles or safety glasses.

12. Remove the mask by holding only the ties. Discard in appropriate waste receptacle.

13. Untie the neck of the gown. Holding only the ties, pull the gown off the shoulders. Pull one arm out of the sleeve, turning the sleeve inside out. Pull the other arm out of the sleeve in the same manner. Be careful the front of the gown does not touch your hands or clothes. Deposit the gown in an appropriate receptacle.

14. Wash hands.

15. Put on lab coat before leaving the area.

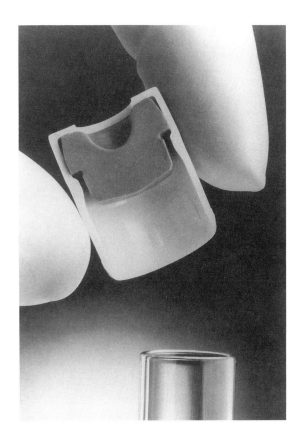

fig 2.4 Vacutainer brand Hemogard tube (courtesy of Becton Dickinson VACUTAINER Systems)

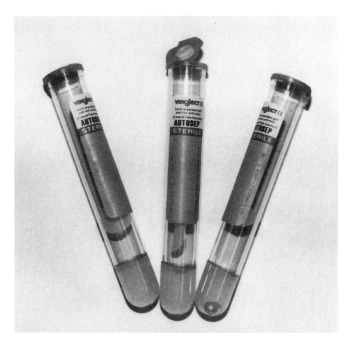

fig 2.5 Peel-off stopper (shown with permission from Terumo Medical Corporation)

lication called the Federal Register. These regulations override any other guidelines issued by any other agency, either government or private.

The entire regulations encompass hundreds of pages. There are points within the regulations that anyone contacting patients or blood and body fluids should be aware of. The OSHA regulations encompass three plans: Exposure Control Plan, Engineering Control Plan, and Work Practice Control Plan.

General Methods of Compliance

Universal Precautions must be observed with blood and body fluids. Hands should be washed with soap and water after any exposure. When handwashing is not available, an appropriate antiseptic cleaner in conjunction with clean cloth/paper towels, or antiseptic towelettes should be used.

Eating, drinking, smoking, applying cosmetics or lip balm, and handling contact lenses are prohibited in work areas. Food and drink must be stored in refrigerators, freezers, and cabinets separate from potentially infectious materials. Food and drink must be consumed in a room separate from the work area, and no contaminated items must enter the room.

All needles and sharps must be placed in containers that are puncture resistant, leakproof, and labeled or color coded as **biohazard**. The biohazard labels must be fluorescent orange or orange-red with lettering or symbols in a contrasting color (Fig. 2.6). The warning labels must also be affixed to containers of regulated waste and to refrigerators or freezers containing blood or other potentially infectious material. Any containers used for transport or storage must also be labeled, and such a container must be of a sealed and leakproof construction. The phlebotomist transporting blood from the patient to the laboratory must use such a container. The required mode of transport is a container so that if the tube containing the blood should break, the blood is contained in the transport container. A number of containers can fill this requirement for transport of specimens within the health care setting. Sealable plastic bags are the most convenient, but sealable plastic containers, paint buckets, or plastic

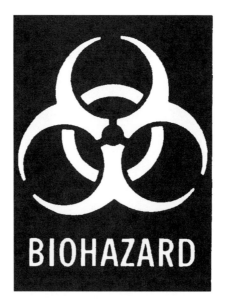

fig 2.6 Biohazard labels

EXERCISE **15** BLOOD COLLECTION IN
AN ISOLATION ROOM

The following procedures are followed to protect the patient or associate from the transmission of disease-causing organisms.

1. Remove all rings, watches, and so on.

2. Prepare to take only essential items into the isolation room. Do not take your tray into the isolation room.

3. Check the isolation card on the door for isolation instructions. This card gives specific information regarding the isolation attire needed.

4. When entering the anteroom, remove three paper towels from the paper towel dispenser. Spread open the paper towels and lay one on top of the other. Place the phlebotomy equipment in the center of the top towel.

5. Wash your hands with soap and water after entering the anteroom. Rinse by letting the water run from the wrists to the fingertips.

6. Dress according to the isolation card instructions. First put on the gown, being careful it does not touch the floor. Put on the mask next, making certain it covers the nose and the mouth.

7. Check to see if a tourniquet and evacuated tube holder are already in the room. Carry the towels with the equipment you will need into the patient's room.

8. Check the patient's armband and draw the specimens according to the required procedure.

9. Discard needles, syringes, and all contaminated equipment in the sharps container. Leave the evacuated tube holder and tourniquet in the room.

10. Open a new alcohol wipe and wipe off the outside of each tube and stopper. Before laying down the cleaned tubes, discard the top paper towel. Now place the tubes on the second towel. Pick up the second towel with the tubes wrapped inside and discard the third (bottom) towel.

11. Carry the tubes and towel into the anteroom.

12. Remove isolation attire in the following order:

    First: Remove one glove. Remove the second glove by inserting your finger under the cuff of the glove and pulling it off over the fingertips. Discard the gloves in the trash receptacle.

    Second: Remove your face mask, touching only the strings.

EXERCISE **15** **BLOOD COLLECTION IN AN ISOLATION ROOM (CONT'D)**

Third: Remove your gown by touching only the inside. Fold the gown so the inside of the gown now faces out and place the gown in the hamper.

13. Wash hands thoroughly.

14. Place tubes, discarding the last towel, in a sealable plastic specimen-transport bag.

EXERCISE **16** **IDENTIFYING SAFETY HAZARDS**

1. Identify any possible safety hazards in the student laboratory.

2. Locate safety equipment in the laboratory (fire extinguishers, fire blankets, eyewash station, spill clean up kit, and so on) and understand how the equipment is used.

buckets with sealable lids can also be used. For transport of potentially infectious materials through the mail, a separate set of standards are used by the postal service.

Material-Safety Data Sheets

The clinical laboratory contains a large array of hazards, ranging from the previously mentioned biological hazards to chemical and electrical hazards. Awareness of chemical hazards has been the focus of OSHA since 1987, when Material-Safety Data Sheets (MSDS) were first introduced under the Hazard Communication Act. The Material-Safety Data Sheets are information sheets that must be kept on file indicating the hazards of the chemicals used in each section of the laboratory. Chemicals used in the laboratory must also carry labels identifying the chemical and showing warnings appropriate for employee protection. This Hazard Communication Act is better known as the "Right to Know" law.

Hazard Identification

Hazards can be identified on the container by a hazard emblem designed by the National Fire Protection Association (Fig. 2.7). The system consists of a diamond-shaped diagram further subdivided into smaller diamonds. "Health hazards" are identified at the left, "flammability" at the top, and "reactivity" at the right. The bottom space is used to identify other hazards or to alert fire-fighting personnel to the possible hazard of using water.

EXERCISE **17** HAZARDOUS CHEMICALS

1. Identify how many hazardous chemicals are in the student laboratory.

2. Examine the labels on the chemicals to determine the severity of the hazard.

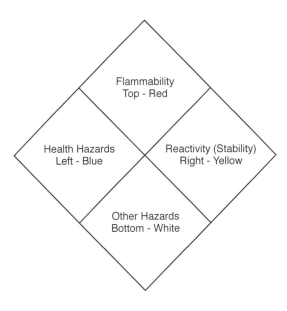

fig **2.7** Hazard identification system

If a spill or splatter of a **hazardous chemical** does occur, eyewash, and showers should be nearby. The shower will "dump" water on the person to dilute the chemical. The eyewash flows water up into the eye. A person using the eyewash will need help in holding the eye open and removing a contact lens if present. The eye should be washed continuously for 15 minutes, and then the person should be taken for treatment.

───────────────────────────────────── **Fire Safety**

Fire safety is taught periodically by each institution. Fire escape routes and your responsibility in a fire are specific to your institution. Fire extinguishers used in a fire are classified according to the type of fire they are to be used on:

Class A: Combustible materials, wood, or paper.

Class B: Flammable liquids and gasses

Class C: Electrical equipment

Class D: Combustible and reactive metals

Most fire extinguishers found in the laboratory are of a universal ABC type.

Radiation Exposure

Phlebotomists are likely to be exposed to radiation. Radiation is present in departments of nuclear medicine and radiology, the radioimmunoassay (RIA) section of the chemistry laboratory, and in patients with radioactive implants. A phlebotomist who encounters the radiation hazard symbol (Fig. 2.8) must be aware of the institution's radiation safety procedures. Most procedures limit exposure by limiting the time the phlebotomist is exposed. The phlebotomist may need to be shielded with a special apron or cover gown. The only other method of protection is staying away from the radiation hazard.

DISPOSAL OF USED MATERIALS

Disposal of potentially infectious materials is controlled by state laws more than by federal regulations. General requirements are standard in most states. A health care institution cannot just set the trash out on the curb and wait for the garbage truck to pick it up.

There are two requirements of disposal of medical waste. First the product must be altered so no one can remove used needles, syringes, or other devices for their own personal use or be injured by an exposed sharp. Second, the waste must be rendered noninfectious

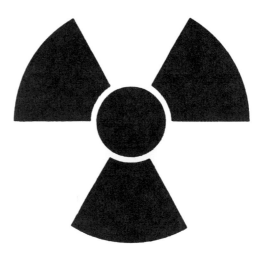

fig `2.8` Universal radiation hazard label

EXERCISE `18` DISPOSAL

1. Identify how the infectious materials in the student laboratory are separated from the the other trash.
2. How is the infectious material disposed of?

EXERCISE 19 ACCIDENTAL NEEDLE STICK

Role-play a situation in which the instructor is the supervisor and the student is a phlebotomist who just experienced an accidental needle stick.

1. Clean the site with soap and water. Make the site continue to bleed. Once bleeding has stopped, clean with alcohol and bandage the injury.

2. Inform the supervisor of the incident.

3. Fill out an incident report form (Fig. 2.9). The phlebotomist's name, date, and time of incident should be entered onto the incident report form. Describe the accident, indicating where it occurred, how it happened, and what part of the body was injured with the stick. Obtain patient's name, medical record number, and birthdate, and enter this on the incident report form.

4. Contact the personnel health department of the hospital. If after office hours, contact the emergency department or designated individual (nursing supervisor).

5. Obtain HIV consent from patient. Many states require the patient to give written consent before the patient can be tested for HIV. Usually the personnel health department or the nursing unit takes care of this detail.

6. The health care worker also needs to give consent for HIV testing and have blood drawn.

7. The patient and associate are screened for HIV, syphilis, and hepatitis. Immunizations are given if necessary.

8. AZT (zidovudine) is offered to associates after an exposure such as contaminated needle stick or laceration. AZT should be considered if:

    a. the associate has been exposed to an AIDS patient or HIV positive patient,

    b. the patient has a high-risk history (drug abuse), or

    c. the source is unknown (needle in trash, for example).

so that anyone handling it will not become infected and the environment will not be contaminated. Three methods of disposal meet these requirements:

1 Incineration
2 Chemical treatment
3 Autoclaving

CONFIDENTIAL REPORT OF EMPLOYEE/VOLUNTEER INCIDENT IN PREPARATION FOR LITIGATION
(Not part of Personnel of Medical Record)

Employee/
Volunteer Involved _____

Department of
Employee/Volunteer _____

Occupation _____

Day of Incident (Circle One)   S   M   Tu   W   Th   F   S

For Hospital Use Only	NURSES STATION	SEX	AGE	STATUS	INCIDENT DATE	REPORT DATE	INCIDENT SHIFT TIME	HOSPITAL CODE NOS.
		____-F ____-M		____Full Time ____Part Time	Mo. Day Year / /	Mo. Day Year / /	___-1st ___-2nd ___AM ___-3rd ___PM	__ __ - __ __ __

CHECK THE APPROPRIATE BOX IN EACH SECTION

WHAT HAPPENED?
- ☐ Handled Patient
- ☐ Handled Object
- ☐ Bumped Against Object
- ☐ Struck by Object
- ☐ Rubbed/Scraped by Object
- ☐ Caught in or Between Object(s)
- ☐ Foreign Particle/Substance Entered Eye(s)
- ☐ Unknown/Other (Specify): _____

CAME IN CONTACT WITH:
- ☐ Sharp Object (Other than needle)
- ☐ Needle or Syringe
- ☐ Electric Current
- ☐ Hot Surface
- ☐ Caustic or Acid

FELL:
- ☐ On Same Level
- ☐ To Different Level

INVOLVED IN:
- ☐ Altercation
- ☐ Motor Vehicle Incident

EXPOSED TO:
- ☐ Radiation
- ☐ Contagious/Infectious Disease
- ☐ Gas, Dust Vapor, Smoke
- ☐ Temperature Extremes

WHAT TYPE OF INJURY / ILLNESS RESULTED?
- ☐ No Injury Apparent
- ☐ Amputation
- ☐ Asphyxiation/Strangulation/ Drowning
- ☐ Burn or Scald
- ☐ Concussion
- ☐ Conjuntivitis (Eye)
- ☐ Unknown/Other (Specify): _____

- ☐ Confusion
- ☐ Laceration-Open Wound
- ☐ Puncture
- ☐ Death
- ☐ Dermatitis
- ☐ Strain/Sprain

- ☐ Inflammation of Joints Tendons, Muscles
- ☐ Dislocation
- ☐ Electrical Shock/Electrocution
- ☐ Fracture
- ☐ Trauma to Eye(s)
- ☐ Frostbite/Freezing

- ☐ Heat Exhaustion or Stroke
- ☐ Hernia/Rupture
- ☐ Hepatitis
- ☐ Disease (Other than Hepatitis)
- ☐ Scratches/Abrasions
- ☐ Multiple Injuries

INDICATE BODY PART AFFECTED:
- ☐ No Body Part Affected
- ☐ Head
- ☐ Face
- ☐ Nose and/or Throat
- ☐ Ear(s)
- ☐ Jaw
- ☐ Mouth/Teeth
- ☐ Neck
- ☐ Unknown/Other (Specify): _____

- ☐ Shoulder
- ☐ Upper Arm
- ☐ Elbow
- ☐ Forearm
- ☐ Wrist
- ☐ Hand
- ☐ Finger(s)

- ☐ Chest
- ☐ Back
- ☐ Abdomen
- ☐ Genitals
- ☐ Hip
- ☐ Upper Leg
- ☐ Knee
- ☐ Lower Leg

- ☐ Ankle
- ☐ Foot/Feet
- ☐ Toe(s)
- ☐ Circulatory System
- ☐ Digestive System
- ☐ Nervous System
- ☐ Respiratory System
- ☐ Multiple Body Parts

WHERE DID IT OCCUR?
- ☐ Patient's Room
- ☐ Patient's Bathroom
- ☐ Other Bathroom
- ☐ Hallway
- ☐ Stairs
- ☐ Nurse's Station
- ☐ Special Care Unit
- ☐ Unknown/Other (Specify): _____

- ☐ Operating Room
- ☐ Obstetrics
- ☐ Pediatrics
- ☐ Laboratory
- ☐ Nursery/Neonatal
- ☐ Physical Therapy
- ☐ Occupational Therapy
- ☐ Respiratory Therapy

- ☐ Psychiatric Area
- ☐ Emergency Room
- ☐ Labor and Delivery
- ☐ Pharmacy
- ☐ Radiology/Nuclear Medicine
- ☐ Cafeteria/Kitchen
- ☐ Office
- ☐ Elevator

- ☐ Lobby/Entrance
- ☐ Walks/Grounds
- ☐ Parking Area
- ☐ Central Supply
- ☐ Storage Area
- ☐ Loading Dock
- ☐ Off Premises
- ☐ Doctor's or Professional Bldg.

WHAT OBJECT WAS INVOLVED?
- ☐ Needle/Syringe
- ☐ Sharps (Other than Needle/Syringe)
- ☐ Bed
- ☐ Wheelchair
- ☐ Patient Handling Equipment
- ☐ Patient/Visitor
- ☐ Unknown/Other (Specify): _____

- ☐ Drugs/Medicines
- ☐ Floor/Floor Surface
- ☐ Scrap, Debris, Waste, etc.
- ☐ Infectious Waste
- ☐ Clothing Apparel, etc.
- ☐ Furniture

- ☐ Machine, Instrument, Tool
- ☐ Liquid NOC
- ☐ Hot Liquid/Steam, etc.
- ☐ Hot Surface
- ☐ Flame, Fire, Smoke
- ☐ Chemical

- ☐ Soaps/Detergents
- ☐ Food or Food Particles
- ☐ Ladder/Step stool
- ☐ Laboratory Animal
- ☐ Building or Structure
- ☐ Vehicle

Person(s) at Scene of Accident: _____

Comments: _____

Supervisor's Signature _____

(Use reverse side if necessary)

fig 2.9 Incident report form

The most common method of disposal of infectious waste is incineration. The waste is burned to an ash, and the ash is taken to the municipal disposal area. This method kills any potentially infectious organisms and makes the items within the waste unusable. Most large hospitals have incinerators to destroy waste and generate steam as a by-product. Special containers should be established for infectious waste, just as there are special disposal containers for sharps.

IMPORTANCE OF FOLLOWING SAFETY GUIDELINES

More important than money is the health care worker's own health. A special exposure procedure must be followed after any exposure from needle stick or splash.

SUMMARY

Universal Precautions apply to all patients. Any patient has the potential to be infected with blood-borne pathogens such as hepatitis or HIV. Following proper blood and body-fluid precautions can nearly eliminate the threat of a health care associate being infected with hepatitis or HIV by a patient. All health care associates should routinely use appropriate barrier precautions to prevent skin and mucous membrane exposure when a possibility exists of contact with blood or other body fluids. Hands and other skin surfaces must be washed immediately after gloves are removed. All health care associates should take precautions to prevent injuries from needles, scalpels, and other sharp instruments. Needles must never be recapped, bent, cut, or broken. Needles, or syringes with needles attached, should not be manipulated by hand unless no alternative exists.

The phlebotomist must also have a knowledge of fire safety, chemical safety, and MSDS sheets. If an accident does occur, the phlebotomist must know the proper procedure to follow.

REVIEW QUESTIONS

Choose the one best answer.

1 The single most important way to prevent the spread of infection in a hospital or other facility is:
a. gowning and gloving
b. handwashing
c. always wearing masks
d. avoiding breathing on patients

2 All of the following are components in the chain of infection *except:*
a. source
b. mode of transportation
c. proper isolation technique
d. susceptible host

3 When a patient develops an infection during hospitalization that was not present upon admission, the infection is classified as:
a. nosocomial
b. communicable
c. infectious
d. unavoidable

4 The primary purpose of infection control is to:
a. determine the source of communicable disease
b. isolate patients from other patients and visitors
c. protect the patient from outside contamination
d. prevent the spread of infection within hospitals and other health care facilities

5 Universal Precautions policy states that if there is a possibility of coming into contact with a patient's blood or any other body fluid, you must wear:
a. a gown
b. goggles
c. gloves
d. nothing, but wash hands immediately

6 According to Universal Precautions, blood and body fluids from which group are considered biohazardous?
a. intravenous drug users
b. homosexuals
c. HIV-positive patients
d. all blood and body fluids

7 Under Universal Precautions, all used needles are to be disposed of in the following manner:
a. recapped
b. discarded intact
c. bent
d. broken or cut off

FURTHER ACTIVITIES

Contact the infection control nurse in a local hospital.

Determine what nosocomial infections are problematic in the facility.

Research how the local hospital prevents the spread of nosocomial infections.

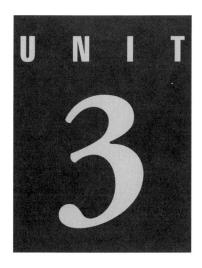

Phlebotomy Equipment

LEARNING OBJECTIVES

After studying this unit, it is the responsibility of the student to know the following objectives:

- Describe the basic units of the metric system.

- State the relationship between bore size and the gauge of a needle.

- Explain the principle of the evacuated system.

- State the manner in which anticoagulants prevent coagulation.

- Name the anticoagulant associated with color-coded tubes.

- State the purpose of additives.

GLOSSARY

Additive	Any material placed in a tube that maintains or facilitates the integrity and function of the specimen.
Thixotropic Separator Gel	A gel material capable of forming an interface between the cells and fluid portion of the blood as a result of centrifugation.
Tourniquet	Any constrictor used to facilitate vein prominence.

INTRODUCTION

Understanding phlebotomy requires knowledge of the metric system. Also required is knowledge of how syringes and evacuated systems are utilized in drawing blood. Anticoagulants are used to provide the best possible specimen for the test the physician needs. Drawing tubes with the correct anticoagulant will provide the specimen needed.

THE METRIC SYSTEM

The metric system is a group of units used to make measurements, for example, of length, volume, temperature, weight, and time. Knowledge of the metric system is necessary to function in the health care setting. Most metric units have a prefix that tells the relationship of that unit to the basic unit. These prefixes are the same throughout the metric system and help to simplify the system. Latin prefixes show divisions of the basic units. For example, *centi* means one-hundredth and *milli* means one-thousandth of the basic unit. Greek prefixes show multiples of the basic unit. For example, *hecto* means 100 times, *kilo* means 1,000 times, and *mega* means 1,000,000 times. The metric system is summarized in Table 3.1.

SYRINGES AND NEEDLES

All methods of venipuncture require the invasive procedure of opening a vein to obtain a blood sample. The syringe-and-needle method is one of the oldest methods known that does not destroy the integrity of the vein. Syringes are made of either glass or plastic; most are plastic. The barrel and plunger (Fig. 3.1) can vary in volume from 1 milliliter to 50 milliliters. The barrel of the syringe is graduated into milliliters.

Pulling on the plunger creates a vacuum within the barrel. The larger the syringe, the greater the amount of vacuum obtained. Too large a vacuum tends to pull too hard on the vein and causes it to collapse. Pulling the plunger slowly and resting between pulls to allow the vein time to refill with blood will prevent collapse of the vein. In general, syringes are used in "difficult-to-draw" patients that have fragile, thin, or "rolly" veins that tend to collapse when an evacuated system is used. Pediatric or geriatric patients typically have such veins. The surface veins on the feet or back of the hands require the syringe technique. The use of a syringe and needle is limited by the capacity of the syringe. The use of a syringe

Table 3–1 Metric System Examples

Length	Volume	Temperature	Weight	Time
Millimeter	Milliliter (or cubic centimeter)	Celsius	Milligram	0 to 2400
Centimeter			Gram	
Meter	Liter		Kilogram	

EXERCISE 20 METRIC SYSTEM

Metric system comparison:

1. Length: Give millimeter measurements for a tumor that would be the size of the top of an evacuated tube.

2. Volume: Measure the amount of blood drawn in milliliters if 1/4 cup of blood is drawn. How many cubic centimeters of blood is this?

3. Temperature: Measure a classmate's body temperature in degrees Celsius.

4. Weight: Measure a person's weight in kilograms.

5. Time: Determine the metric time for 8:00 A.M., 12 noon, 4:00 P.M., 6:00 P.M., and midnight.

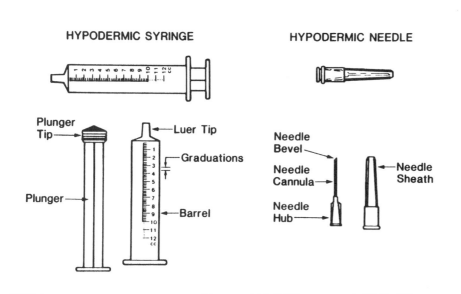

fig 3.1 Syringe and needle

larger than 10 to 15 milliliters is not recommended. If a large amount of blood is needed, a butterfly collection set is to be used. This device is discussed in Unit 4. Syringes are also used in special procedures when blood must be drawn and then transferred to a different container.

The recommended length of the needle is 1 to 1 1/2 inches. The gauges of needles that are used in health care are 25, 23, 22, 21, 20, 18, and 16; the smallest needle is a 25 gauge and the largest a 16 gauge (Table 3.2).

EVACUATED SYSTEM

The evacuated system is often called the Vacutainer system. This can be a misnomer because the term *Vacutainer* is a brand name for the evacuated system carried by a company called Becton Dickinson. Phlebotomists will often say "Vacutainer" when they are using another company's product.

The principle of the evacuated blood collection system is the vacuum created when the plunger of the syringe is pulled. In the evacuated system, a tube with a vacuum already in it attaches to the needle, and the tube's vacuum is replaced by blood. The system consists of a double-pointed needle, a plastic holder or adapter, and a series of vacuum tubes with rubber stoppers (Fig. 3.2).

The key to the evacuated system is the needle. The needle is double pointed with a different length needle on each end and a screw hub near the center. The longer needle has the proper bevel to pierce the skin and enter the vein. The shorter needle pierces the rubber stopper on the evacuated tube. The shorter needle is covered by a rubber sleeve (Fig. 3.3). This sleeve works as a valve that stops the flow of blood when the tube is removed. Pushing the tube into the holder compresses the rubber sleeve and exposes the needle to enter the tube. When the tube is removed, the sleeve slides back over the needle and stops the flow of blood.

The needle can be thought of as a pipeline that is going to deliver blood from the patient to the tube. The blood is pulled out of the patient due to the vacuum of the tube.

The bevel of the needle must always be facing upward when the needle is inserted into the vein. When looking straight down on the needle as the needle is inserted into the skin, the opening in the needle will be visible. The needle should be inserted at a 15° angle to the surface of the skin (Fig. 3.4).

Table **3–2** Needle Gauges

25: smallest gauge needle, often can cause hemolysis of blood.
23: used with butterfly system or with syringes 0 to 5 milliliters in capacity.
22
21: used with evacuated systems.
20
18: large size not often used for phlebotomy.
16: used for blood donation

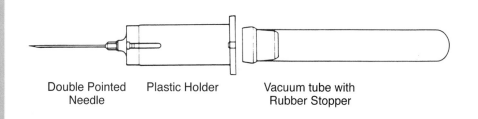

Double Pointed   Plastic Holder   Vacuum tube with
Needle   Rubber Stopper

fig **3.2** Vacutainer system (courtesy of Becton Dickinson VACUTAINER Systems)

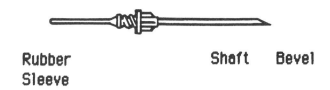

Rubber   **Shaft**   **Bevel**
Sleeve

fig **3.3** Vacutainer needle (courtesy of Becton Dickinson VACUTAINER Systems)

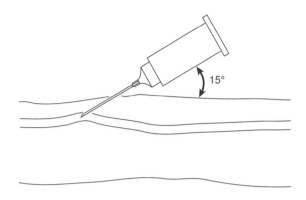

15°

fig **3.4** Proper angle of insertion

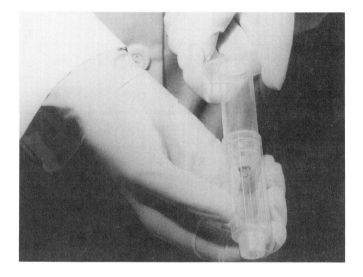

fig **3.5** VACUTAINER brand Safety-Lok Needle Holder (courtesy of Becton Dickinson VACUTAINER Systems)

The holder for the needle makes the task of collecting the blood sample easier. The holder is held in the same manner as you would hold the barrel of a syringe. The holders come in two sizes, one size for adult venipuncture and one size for small-diameter tubes used on pediatric patients. The holders have changed in recent years from the basic holders (Fig. 3.2) to include holders with outer sleeves that slide over the contaminated needle. This outer sleeve protects the phlebotomist from needle sticks until the needle can be disposed of (Fig. 3.5).

ANTICOAGULANTS

Different tests require different types of blood specimens. Some specimens require a serum sample and need to be drawn in a tube that allows the blood to clot. Others require a whole-blood or plasma specimen and must not be allowed to clot. To prevent clotting of the blood, the tube will contain an anticoagulant. An anticoagulant is a chemical substance that prevents coagulation by removing calcium in the form of calcium salts or by inhibiting the conversion of prothrombin to thrombin. Coagulation is a path on which each step must be taken before a clot forms (Table 3.3). If a step is not taken, the blood does not clot.

This process of clotting can be stopped in the test tube. A tube that contains an anticoagulant removes one of the steps, and the blood will not clot. The anticoagulant prevents clotting in a way that depends on the anticoagulant used. The basic anticoagulants used are oxalates, citrates, ethylenediaminetetraacetic acid (EDTA), and heparin (Table 3.4).

Various **additives** are placed in the tubes to improve the quality of the specimen. These additives are not anticoagulants or preservatives but are used to improve specimen quality or to accelerate specimen processing. Some serum tubes have a clot activator that speeds the clotting process. This clot activator consists of silica particles on the sides of the tube that initiate the clotting process.

A type of clot activator that is used for emergency (STAT) testing is thrombin. Thrombin hastens the clotting process faster than the silica particles.

Serum and plasma tubes can also be purchased with a **thixotrophic separator gel** (Fig. 3.6). This gel is an inert material that undergoes a temporary change in viscosity during centrifugation. It has a density that is intermediate to cells/clot and plasma/serum. When centrifuged, the gel moves up the sides of the tube and engulfs the cells/clot; an interface of gel forms that separates the cells/clot from the plasma/serum (Fig. 3.7).

TOURNIQUETS

The **tourniquet** constricts the flow of blood in the arm and makes the veins more prominent. A tourniquet is a soft, pliable, rubber strip approximately 1 inch wide by 15 to 18 inches long. This rubber strip serves as the best tourniquet for all conditions. Velcro strips are also available, and round rubber tubing is occasionally used. The rubber strip is the best because it can easily be released with one hand. Being about 1 inch wide, it does not cut into the patient's arm but distributes the pressure. Tourniquets can be wiped off easily with alcohol to prevent spreading of infection and are inexpensive enough that they can be replaced often (Fig. 3.8).

Table 3–3 Steps to a Clot

1. Uncoagulated blood
2. Calcium utilized
3. Prothrombin converts to thrombin
4. Fibrinogen converts to fibrin
5. Clot forms

Table 3–4   Tube Guide

Tube Color	Additive	Additive Action	Laboratory Use
Gray	Potassium oxalate/ sodium fluoride	Binds calcium Stabilizes glucose values	Glucose test
Blue	Sodium citrate	Binds calcium	Coagulation studies: tubes must be filled to the proper level.
Lavender	Ethylinediamine-diaminetetraacetic acid (EDTA)	Binds calcium	Hematology testing: Complete Blood Count
Green	Lithium heparin Sodium heparin	Inhibits prothrombin to thrombin	Plasma determinations in chemistry
Royal Blue	Sodium heparin	Inhibits prothrombin to thrombin	Plasma toxicology
	No additive	Clot forms	Serum toxicology
Orange	Thrombin	Fast clot formation	State serum determinations
Red	No additive	Clot forms	Serum testing
Special Blue	Thrombin/soybean trypsin inhibitor	Clot forms	Fibrin Degradation Products (FDP)/Fibrin Split Products (FSP)

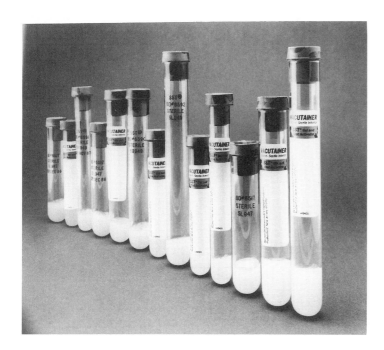

fig 3.6   Separator gel tube (courtesy of Becton Dickinson VACUTAINER Systems)

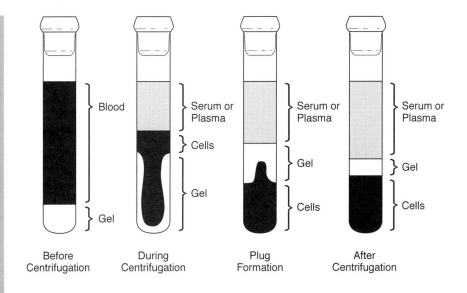

fig 3.7 Separator gel tube: centrifugation process

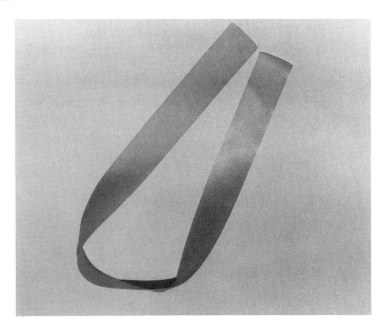

fig 3.8 Tourniquet

SPECIMEN COLLECTION TRAYS

The phlebotomist needs a specimen collection tray to hold all the equipment necessary for proper specimen collection. This tray is taken to the patient's room so that whatever procedure is performed the phlebotomist will be prepared. These trays vary depending on the type of collections usually done, or the type of hospital or laboratory the phlebotomist works at. In some cases, a tray will not be adequate, and the phlebotomist will have a stocked cart to roll from room to room. The tray is usually preferred because it is more portable and can be taken up stairs to avoid a long wait at the elevator. Trays come in a variety of sizes and shapes to fit the phlebotomist's preference and needs (Fig. 3.9).

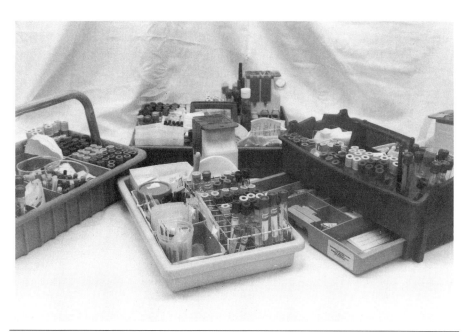

fig **3.9** Phlebotomy trays

E X E R C I S E **21** GEL TUBE

Refer to Exercise 10. Centrifuge five tubes of blood with gel to demonstrate how the gel forms an interface between the cells and the serum/plasma.

1. Centrifuge each tube of blood individually for:
   a. 1 minute
   b. 3 minutes
   c. 5 minutes
   d. 10 minutes
   e. 15 minutes

2. Use the same centrifuge and maintain the same speed for each tube centrifuged.

3. Line the tubes in a test tube rack in the order of time centrifuged.

4. Observe the change in the gel as the centrifuge time increases.

5. In your student notebook, write down the differences in the five tubes and draw pictures of the position of the gel in each tube.

EXERCISE 22 SPECIMEN COLLECTION TRAYS

Borrow from a hospital laboratory several types of trays used for blood collection. Divide the class into four groups. Each group meets and reports to the class on dangers that are possible on a specimen collection tray.

SUMMARY

The metric system is the system of measurement used in health care. This system is used to measure syringes and evacuated systems. Blood specimens are collected in tubes that contain an anticoagulant or have no additive. This produces whole blood, plasma, or serum specimens. The test that is ordered dictates the type of specimen the phlebotomist must collect.

REVIEW QUESTIONS

Choose the one best answer.

1 10 milliliter (ml) is the same as:
a. 1 liter
b. 10 deciliters
c. 10 cubic centimeters (cc)
d. none of the above

2 The bore of a needle that is the smallest is:
a. 16 gauge needle
b. 20 gauge needle
c. 21 gauge needle
d. 23 gauge needle

3 Which of the following anticoagulants prevent coagulation of the blood by removing calcium through the formation of insoluble calcium salts?
a. EDTA
b. oxalate
c. sodium citrate
d. heparin
e. all the above
f. a, b, and c

4 An anticoagulant is an additive placed in an evacuated tube in order to:
a. dilute the blood prior to testing
b. ensure the sterility of the tube
c. make the blood clot faster
d. prevent the blood from clotting

5 A green stoppered evacuated tube contains what kind of anticoagulant?
a. citrate
b. fluoride
c. heparin
d. no additive

FURTHER ACTIVITIES

Contact several evacuated tube companies for catalogues to determine the different types of evacuated tubes that are available.

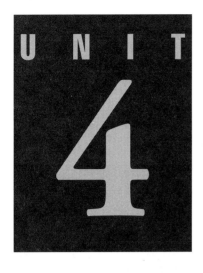

Phlebotomy Technique

LEARNING OBJECTIVES

After studying this unit, it is the responsibility of the student to know the following objectives:

■ Explain the three skills used in collecting blood.

■ Explain the importance of correct patient identification, complete specimen labeling, and proper accessioning.

■ Explain how a tourniquet makes the veins more prominent

■ Describe the step-by-step procedure for drawing blood with a syringe, evacuated system, or butterfly.

■ Explain how to handle different patient reactions to venipuncture.

■ Discuss the three blood-collection alternatives when a patient has an IV running in one arm.

■ Describe the proper technique for drawing from an indwelling line.

■ Describe the Allen test.

■ Explain the proper procedure for handling arterial blood.

GLOSSARY

Aliquot	Part of the whole specimen that has been taken off for use or storage.
Cannula	Device used for access for dialyzing and for drawing blood in kidney patients.

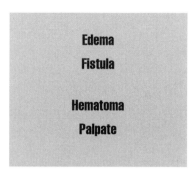

Edema	Abnormal accumulation of fluid in the tissues resulting in swelling.
Fistula	Artificial shunt connection done by surgical procedure to fuse the vein and artery together. Used for dialysis only.
Hematoma	Leakage of blood out of the vein during or after venipuncture that causes a bruise.
Palpate	To search for a vein with a pressure-and-release touch.

I N T R O D U C T I O N

Correct venipuncture of a patient requires the phlebotomist to have a knowledge of each detail of the venipuncture procedure. The phlebotomist uses a variety of skills and techniques to obtain the best specimen. Unless all the venipuncture steps are followed, the quality of the specimen and the safety of the phlebotomist will be compromised.

STEPS IN THE BLOOD-COLLECTION TECHNIQUE

Venipuncture procedure is a detailed procedure; certain steps must be taken for each venipuncture (Table 4.1).

Table **4–1** Steps in Venipuncture

1. Prepare accessioning order for the patient.
2. Identify patient.
3. Verify diet/drug restrictions.
4. Assemble supplies and inspect equipment.
5. Reassure the patient.
6. Position the patient.
7. Verify paperwork and tubes.
8. Perform venipuncture.
9. Fill the tubes (if syringe and needle are used).
10. Bandage patient's arm.
11. Dispose of sharps in proper container.
12. Label tubes.
13. Chill specimen (only for certain tests).
14. Eliminate diet restrictions.
15. Time-stamp or computer-verify paperwork.
16. Send correctly labeled tubes to proper laboratory departments.

APPROACHING THE PATIENT

The phlebotomist uses three skills when contacting patients for phlebotomy:

1 Social skill

2 Clerical skill

3 Technical skill

Social skills are important. Patients are often angry about their condition and take it out on the first person they see. The phlebotomist could just be waking them up or could be entering the room right after the doctor gave them bad news. Whatever a patient says, it is inappropriate to counter with unprofessional remarks. The easiest way to defuse an upset patient is to be as polite as possible and explain that the doctor's orders need to be carried out.

The phlebotomist is the laboratory representative. The patient's response to how well the laboratory performed while the patient was in the hospital is not influenced by the sophisticated instrumentation used to test the specimens. The response to friends and neighbors could be, "The blood drawers were the best I had ever seen. They were polite, skilled, and very gentle." The finest social skill guarantees this response from each patient.

The phlebotomist's social skills will also be put to the test when a patient refuses to have blood drawn.

Clerical skills are used constantly, and their misuse contributes to the most errors in the health care setting. For the phlebotomist, the clerical skill is as simple as drawing the correct patient's blood and labeling it with the correct name.

Technical skills mean obtaining blood successfully with minimal pain. They consist of whatever method is used to complete the procedure: venipuncture, arterial sample, or microcollections through skin puncture.

Patient and Specimen Identification

Proper patient and specimen identification are essential to accurate patient testing. The results of sample testing will be wrong if the sample is not accurately identified. Most patients have a hospital identification bracelet that includes their first and last names, hospital numbers (often there are two sets of numbers), birthdate, and physician. The phlebotomist, on entering a room, should not say, "Mr. Jones, I'm here to draw your blood," assuming if the patient says "yes" that he is Mr. Jones. The patient will often have

---

E X E R C I S E 23 SOCIAL SKILL

Two students from the class join in a role play in front of class.

1. One student plays the phlebotomist with an order to draw a patient's blood sample at 3:00 A.M.

2. The other student plays the role of the patient who has to be awakened from a deep sleep.

EXERCISE   24   PATIENT REFUSAL

Two students from the class join in a role play in front of class.

1. One student plays the phlebotomist with an order to draw a patient's blood.
2. The other student plays the role of the patient who refuses to have blood drawn.

EXERCISE   25   CLERICAL SKILL

Two students from the class join in a role play in front of class.

1. One student plays the phlebotomist with an order to draw a patient's blood sample.
2. The other student plays the role of the patient who is not the same patient the phlebotomist is to draw.
3. Does the phlebotomist determine this is the incorrect patient?
4. If the phlebotomist did determine this was the incorrect patient, how was this accomplished?

been asleep or not paying attention and will answer "yes" no matter what the circumstance. Ask the conscious patient to state his or her full name. This both lets the patient realize someone is in the room and gets the patient thinking so that he or she will be awake when blood is collected. The phlebotomist still needs to check the armband to verify the correct patient's blood is being drawn even after the patient has stated his or her name. In addition to checking the patient's name, check the patient's identification numbers.

The identification numbers on the patient's armband are compared to the name and numbers on the order form used in the health care institution. These order forms can be a manual requisition that is usually a multipart carbon form (Fig. 4.1) or an adhesive computer label (Fig. 4.2). The manual requisition is usually imprinted from an addressograph plate that prints the patient's name, identification numbers, physician, and room number. This plate is similar to a credit card plate, except that it contains more information. The manual requisition can also be handwritten.

The computer label has several advantages in being able to list the specific test that was

EXERCISE 26 MANUAL TUBE LABELLING

Each student from the class is to label an empty evacuated tube as if he or she were the patient. Use the following information:

1. Patient's complete first and last names.

2. Hospital registration number(s) (use your social security number).

3. Room number (use classroom number).

4. Date and time of draw.

5. Phlebotomist's initials.

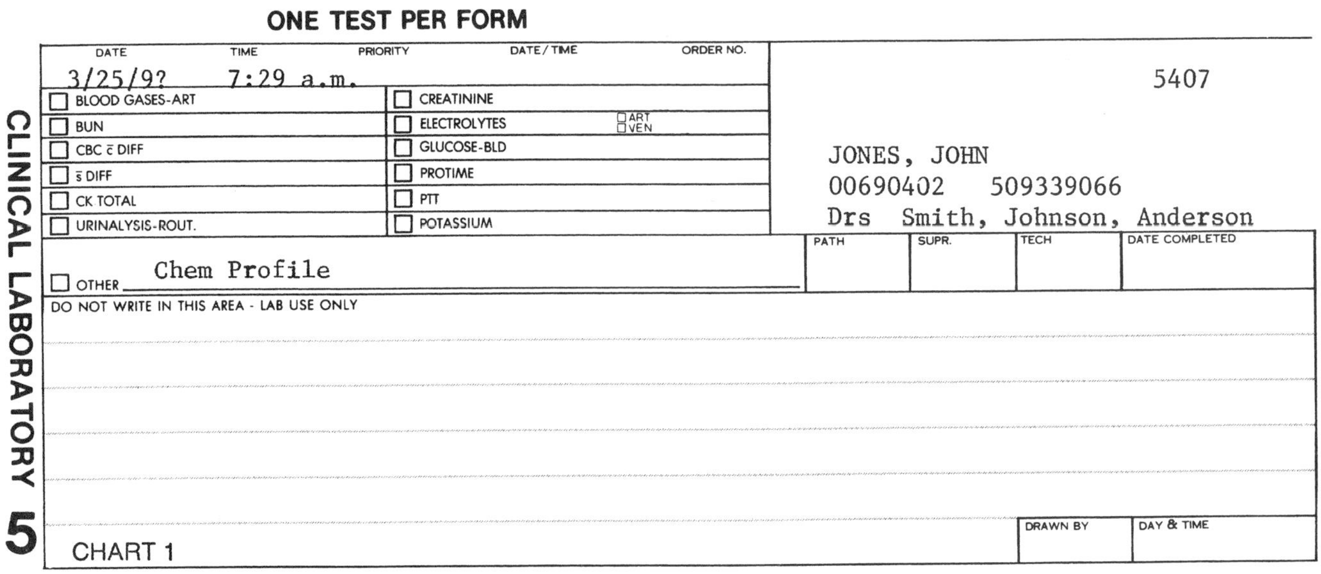

ONE TEST PER FORM

DATE	TIME	PRIORITY	DATE / TIME	ORDER NO.		
3/25/9?	7:29 a.m.					5407

☐ BLOOD GASES-ART	☐ CREATININE
☐ BUN	☐ ELECTROLYTES ☐ ART ☐ VEN
☐ CBC c̄ DIFF	☐ GLUCOSE-BLD
☐ s̄ DIFF	☐ PROTIME
☐ CK TOTAL	☐ PTT
☐ URINALYSIS-ROUT.	☐ POTASSIUM

JONES, JOHN
00690402   509339066
Drs Smith, Johnson, Anderson

PATH	SUPR.	TECH	DATE COMPLETED

☐ OTHER ___Chem Profile___

DO NOT WRITE IN THIS AREA - LAB USE ONLY

CLINICAL LABORATORY 5

CHART 1

DRAWN BY	DAY & TIME

fig 4.1 Manual requisition

ordered and the required specimen and specimen requirements. The label can also be adhesive so it can be attached directly to the tube. Smaller labels can also be printed at the same time for smaller **aliquot** specimens. The computer has many other advantages, in timing the printing of orders, sorting lists of orders for one patient at one time, and speeding entry of draw times and test results. Most hospitals use some type of computer system for ordering tests and reporting results. The computer labels print off in a roll where one label follows the other. Four labels attached as in Fig. 4.2 require special attention. One label must be checked against the other carefully to assure that each label is for the same person, date, and time. Labels may also contain bar codes to assist in electronic patient and sample identification. Identifying patients by the computer labels and assuring each

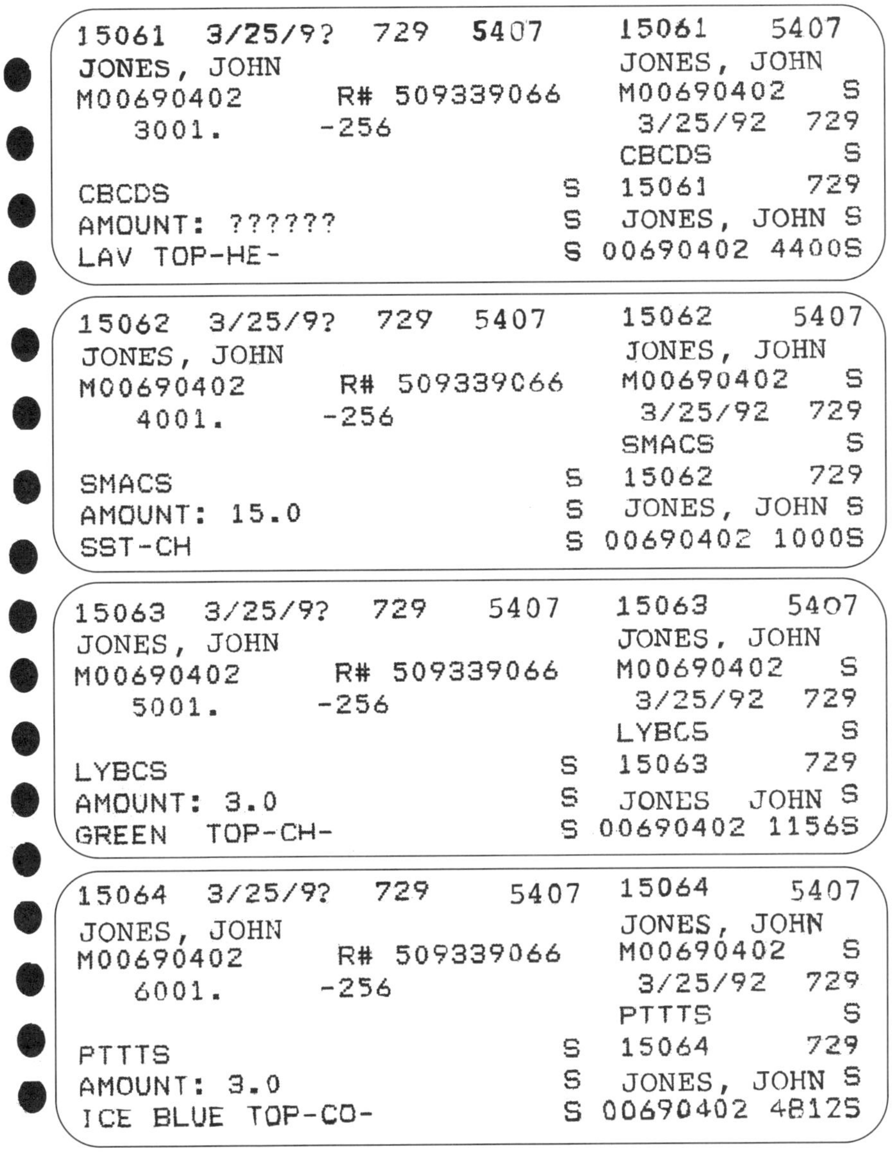

```
15061   3/25/9?   729    5407      15061      5407
JONES, JOHN                        JONES, JOHN
M00690402        R# 509339066      M00690402    S
    3001.        -256                 3/25/92   729
                                    CBCDS        S
CBCDS                         S     15061      729
AMOUNT: ??????                S     JONES, JOHN S
LAV TOP-HE-                   S  00690402 4400S
```

```
15062   3/25/9?   729    5407      15062      5407
JONES, JOHN                        JONES, JOHN
M00690402        R# 509339066      M00690402    S
    4001.        -256                 3/25/92   729
                                    SMACS        S
SMACS                         S     15062      729
AMOUNT: 15.0                  S     JONES, JOHN S
SST-CH                        S  00690402 1000S
```

```
15063   3/25/9?   729    5407      15063      5407
JONES, JOHN                        JONES, JOHN
M00690402        R# 509339066      M00690402    S
    5001.        -256                 3/25/92   729
                                    LYBCS        S
LYBCS                         S     15063      729
AMOUNT: 3.0                   S     JONES  JOHN S
GREEN   TOP-CH-               S  00690402 1156S
```

```
15064   3/25/9?   729    5407      15064      5407
JONES, JOHN                        JONES, JOHN
M00690402        R# 509339066      M00690402    S
    6001.        -256                 3/25/92   729
                                    PTTTS        S
PTTTS                         S     15064      729
AMOUNT: 3.0                   S     JONES, JOHN S
ICE BLUE TOP-CO-              S  00690402 4812S
```

fig 4.2 Computer labels

label used is for that patient requires the use of a specific procedure. With computerized systems, the phlebotomist will verify in the computer when the blood was drawn.

Accessioning Order

Each request for a blood specimen must include a number to identify all paperwork and supplies associated with each patient. This is giving the patient an accessioning order, a unique number that can be used to trace that specimen and patient. This is to ensure accurate and prompt processing of various forms required when a venipuncture is performed and the results are analyzed. The blood request forms should include the information given in Table 4.2.

Outpatient and inpatient specimens are labeled after the specimen is drawn and before

EXERCISE ■27■ PATIENT IDENTIFICATION PROCEDURE

Two students from the class join in a role play.

1. One student has on an armband.

2. The phlebotomist student has four labels and goes through the patient identification procedure.

Procedure:

1. Approach the patient in a professional and courteous manner.

2. Collect all equipment and patient labels needed for only that venipuncture and take to patient's bedside.

3. Use the band identification procedure to ensure proper patient identification.

4. Perform a band identification procedure by doing either a label-to-label check or a band-to-label check.
   a. For a label-to-label check, compare the patient's first and last names and hospital registration number on the first label to those on band to be sure that they are exactly the same. Then compare the first label to each following label.
   b. For a band-to-label check, compare the patient's first and last names and hospital registration number on every label to those on the band.

5. After ensuring that this is the correct patient, perform the venipuncture.

6. Perform band identification a second time using one of the above methods.

7. Read each label as it is attached to the tube before leaving the bedside.

8. If computer labels are unavailable, labeling of the tubes may be done by:
   a. Addressograph labels.
   b. Handwriting the patient's complete first and last names, hospital registration number(s), room number, date, and time of draw as required by the test.

9. Write the first and last initials of the phlebotomist on each specimen label.

10. If the patient does not have an identification band on his/her wrist or ankle, or if the identification band is not correct, notify the nurse or nursing unit secretary. *Do not draw blood unless the patient is wearing a correct identification band.*

11. All three identification checks are required: one verbal name check and two identification band checks.

EXERCISE **27** PATIENT IDENTIFICATION PROCEDURE (CONT'D)

12. If a labeling error is suspected, the supervisor must be notified.

Optional Exercise: The instructor adds errors to the armband or labels. The student is then observed to see if the errors are noticed.

Table 4–2 Blood Request Information

1. Patient's name and age from ID plate or wristband.
2. Identification number.
3. Date and time the specimen is obtained.
4. Name or initials of person who obtains the specimen.
5. Accessioning number.
6. Physician's name.
7. Department for which work is being done.
8. Other useful information, for example, special comments, unusual sampling site, drawn near an IV site.

---

the phlebotomist leaves the patient. Each tube and label must be checked to assure that proper identification is completed.

Positioning the Patient

The position of the patient is critical in proper blood collection. The position should be comfortable for both the patient and the phlebotomist. Proper positioning of the patient will make the patient feel more at ease, and the phlebotomist will be better able to perform the venipuncture.

Selecting the Appropriate Venipuncture Site

The appropriate venipuncture site can vary depending on the patient. The usual site that is first checked is the upper region of the arm. The primary vein used in the upper arm is the median cubital vein. This is usually the prominent vein in the middle of the bend of the arm (Fig. 4.3). The basilic, cephalic, or median vein can be used as a second alternative. These veins may be not accessible or may not be prominent enough to obtain a blood sample. The next step is to go to the back of the hand to obtain venous access. The veins in the back of the hand have the tendency to "roll" more than the arm veins because they are not supported by as much tissue and are near the surface. To prevent this, the vein will have to be held in place by the index finger and the thumb while a smaller-gauge needle or a butterfly is used. The hand

EXERCISE 28 UNKNOWN PATIENT IDENTIFICATION

Accessioning a patient in the emergency room where identification is not immediate, it is necessary to:

1. Assign a master identification number (temporary) to the patient. A three-part identification tag with the same master number on all three parts is assigned to the patient:
   a. Attach the first part to the patient's arm.
   b. Attach the second part to the specimen.
   c. Attach the third part to the blood transfusion bag if a transfusion has been ordered.

2. Select the appropriate test forms and write the identification number on the forms.

3. Complete the necessary labels and apply to the specimens

4. Cross-reference the permanent identification number to the temporary number after a permanent number is assigned.

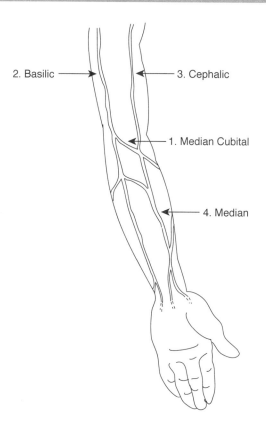

fig **4.3** Veins in the arm

E X E R C I S E ■29■ POSITIONING THE PATIENT

Two students are selected from the class to pair as patient and phlebotomist. Two situations are presented.

1. Patient that does not have a problem with having blood drawn:
    a. The patient must be in a seated or reclined position before any attempt is made to draw blood.
    b. Do not allow the patient to sit on a tall stool or stand while drawing blood. There is always the possibility that the patient will faint (syncope) and be injured.
    c. The sitting position requires a chair with adequate arm supports that are adjustable for the best venipuncture position.

2. Patient that will faint (syncope):
    a. Have the patient lie down whenever a patient indicates he or she is apprehensive and has fainted while having blood draw.
    b. The reclined position is the ideal position from which to draw blood from the patient.
    c. A pillow may be required to help support the patient's arm, keeping it straight for easier venous access.

veins are ideal for a 3- to 5-milliliter syringe with a 22-gauge needle. A careful, slow pull on the syringe will obtain the blood sample without collapsing the vein or hemolyzing the blood. The wrist veins are also an alternative but generally are much more painful than the other sites. The foot and ankle veins may also be used if the patient's physician gives permission to use them. The veins in the foot or ankle will also have the tendency to "roll."

The order for checking for the best available site is (1) upper arm, (2) hand, (3) wrist, and (4) ankle or foot. The next alternative is for a more experienced phlebotomist to check, or if possible, to draw the sample from a fingerstick.

A tourniquet must be used to assist the phlebotomist in feeling a vein. The tourniquet is applied 3 to 4 inches above the puncture site. It is applied tight enough to stop the flow of blood in the veins but not to prevent the flow of blood in the arteries. This is very similar to damming a small stream. When a stream is dammed, the water will form a pond in front of the dam. With the tourniquet applied, the arteries will fill the veins with blood, pooling the blood in the veins before the tourniquet. This pooling of blood makes the veins more prominent. The veins can then be **palpated** to determine their direction, depth, and size. The tourniquet should be on the arm no longer than 1 minute. Just as a stream will become stagnant when it no longer flows, a tourniquet that is left on too long will cause hemoconcentration of the blood and an increased concentration of constituents in the blood sample.

The tourniquet should ideally be removed as soon as blood flow is established. This is not practical for the beginning phlebotomist, for whom the act of removing the tourniquet moves the needle and/or vein just enough so that no more blood can be obtained and the

EXERCISE **30** VENIPUNCTURE SITES

The students in the class each find a partner. One plays the phlebotomist and the other the patient. When the exercise is completed the roles are reversed.

1. Wrap the tourniquet around the arm 3 to 4 inches above the venipuncture site (Fig. 4.4).

2. While holding the ends tight, tuck one portion of the end under the other (Fig. 4.5).

3. Check that the tourniquet will not come loose. The ends of the tourniquet should be pointed upward (Fig. 4.6).

4. The phlebotomist feels for a vein that would be acceptable to draw blood from (Fig. 4.7).

5. The instructor is asked to check the site for acceptability.

6. Patients that have unusual sites or are special challenges are shared with the class.

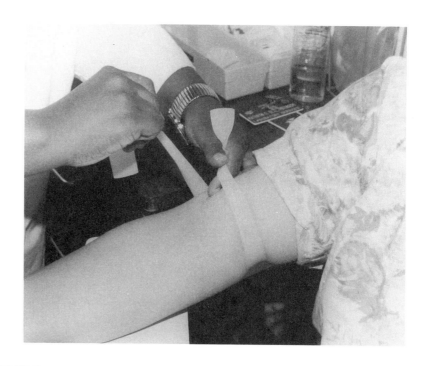

fig 4.4 Wrap the tourniquet around the arm 3 to 4 inches above the venipuncture site

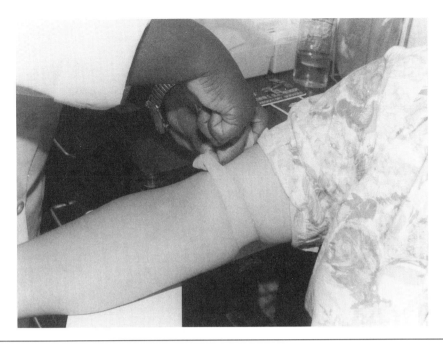

fig **4.5** While holding the ends tight, tuck one portion of the end under the other

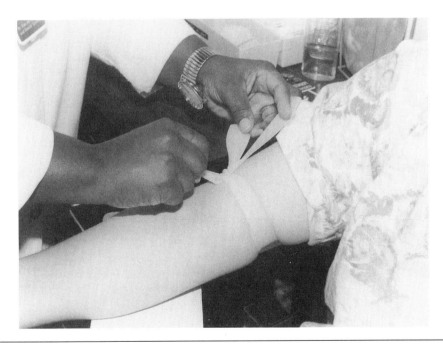

fig **4.6** Check that the tourniquet will not come loose. The ends of the tourniquet should be pointed upward

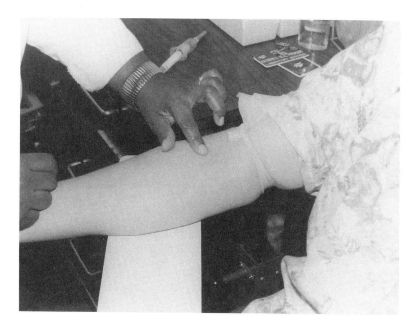

fig 4.7 Feel for a vein

patient's blood has to be redrawn. It is recommended to wait to remove the tourniquet until just before the needle is removed from the patient. Not removing the tourniquet before the needle is removed causes blood to be forced out of the needle hole and into the surrounding skin, resulting in a **hematoma**.

Performing a Safe Venipuncture

The first step in collecting a venous blood sample is to find the site that will give the best blood return. The vein must be felt for with the tip of the index finger. Palpate and trace the path of the vein several times. Avoid using the thumb because it has a pulse and is not as sensitive as the rest of the fingers. The vein will feel soft and bouncy to the touch. The roundness and the direction that the vein follows will be determined. Not all veins go straight up and down the arm. If no veins become prominent, retie the tourniquet tighter, but not so tight as to stop the flow of arterial blood into the arm.

If the "vein" that is felt has a pulsing action to it, this indicates an artery in the patient's arm and should not be punctured. Tendons will also be deceptive and appear to be a vein. They do not have the soft bouncy feel and will be hard to the touch. Puncturing a tendon gives no blood return and is painful to the patient. Nerves also run the length of the arm. The nerves can not be seen or felt, but by avoiding deep probing venipunctures, the chance of touching a nerve is diminished. If the patient complains about the venipuncture hurting excessively, it is best to stop and try another site.

Veins of **edematous** arms that are swollen due to fluid in the tissue will not be prominent and the tourniquet will not be effective due to the swelling. Placement of the tourniquet has the potential for tissue damage and leaves a temporary indentation in the arm. Areas of scarring are also to be avoided due to possible injury or excessive pain to the patient. Specimens collected from a hematoma area may cause erroneous test results. If another vein site is not available, the specimen is collected distal from the hematoma. Because of the potential for harm to the patient due to lymphostasis, the arm on the side of a masectomy should be avoided. If the patient has had a double masectomy, a physician should be consulted prior to drawing the blood.

Before a venipuncture can be performed, all supplies and equipment must be assembled. It is best to prepare everything before greeting the patient. As the patient's blood is drawn, be able to reach the tubes needed without crossing over the patient or stretching and possibly moving the needle after it is in the patient. Remember that a tube occasionally will not fill all the way; in this case it is best to keep a few spare tubes or have the phlebotomy tray within reach. Now it is time to greet the patient.

SYRINGE SPECIMEN COLLECTION

The patient has been identified, paperwork and tubes verified, equipment assembled, and the patient is in a comfortable position. The next step is to tie the tourniquet. Have the patient close his or her hand and then select a vein. Place the patient's arm in a downward position if possible. After location of an acceptable vein, mentally map the location. Set mental crosshairs on it by visualizing the puncture site. It might be slightly over from this freckle and a little down from that wrinkle. Set those mental crosshairs for an accurate puncture. Now the site needs to be cleaned with a gauze pad soaked with 70 percent isopropyl alcohol solution. A commercially prepared alcohol pad, or chlorhexidine, 0.5 percent, in alcohol may also be used. The skin is cleansed in a circular motion from the center to the outside. The area is allowed to air dry to prevent hemolysis of the specimen and to prevent the patient from feeling a burning sensation during phlebotomy.

E X E R C I S E **GREETING THE PATIENT**

Two students from the class join in a role play in front of class. One student plays the phlebotomist, the other, the patient.

1. The patient must be reassured that the procedure is going to be simple and there will be only a slight inconvenience.
2. Be friendly and outgoing, and talk to the patient, explaining the procedure.
3. Do not tell the patient this is not going to hurt.
4. The anticipation of having blood drawn is worse to many patients than the actual draw.
5. Polite conversation with all patients gives them the feeling someone cares about them.
6. This concern for the patient will continue to bring patients back to that health care institution.
7. At the end of the role play the rest of the class analyzes the performance to determine where improvements could be made.
8. The class then determines what was good and should not be changed.

While the alcohol is drying, put on gloves if you have not already done so. Some authorities suggest gloves be put on before you feel for the vein. This is required for the patient in isolation. For the normal, unisolated patient, the gloves are not needed until there is a chance of coming in contact with blood and body fluid. The main deterrent to a phlebotomist wearing gloves is the inability to "feel" the vein. The time it takes for the alcohol to air dry on the arm is just enough time to put on gloves. To avoid forgetting where the collection site is, palpate the vein 1 to 2 inches above and below the intended puncture site. This helps the phlebotomist feel that the vein is located in a straight line, and these points can be used to "reset" the mental crosshairs without contaminating the venipuncture site.

The syringe technique is not used as much as the evacuated system is used. The techniques developed in the syringe method are building blocks for the evacuated tube technique and all other techniques.

The syringe is ideal for taking small blood samples from fragile surface veins or veins in the back of the hand. A detailed procedure for venipuncture with syringe is as follows (outlined in Exercise 33):

When a syringe is used, the blood obtained must be placed in appropriate containers. To place the blood in evacuated tubes, puncture the stopper with the syringe needle and allow blood to enter the tube until the flow stops. The rubber stoppers must not be removed. Running blood down the side of the tube after removing the stopper is not recommended because aerosols and splattering of blood can occur. Mix if any anticoagulant is present. Do not hold the tube in your hand as you puncture the stopper. There is the potential for missing the stopper or slipping off the stopper and puncturing yourself. The best method is to have the tubes in a test tube rack and then puncture the tubes using only

EXERCISE **32** **PROPER HAND POSITION TO HOLD A SYRINGE**

The instructor gives each student a syringe and needle.

1. Attach the needle to the syringe.
2. Hold the syringe and needle system in your dominant hand and cradled on the four fingers.
3. The thumb is then placed on top of the syringe.
4. A right-handed person holds the syringe in the right hand, leaving the left hand to pull on the plunger. A left-handed person does the opposite.
5. With the syringe held in this position, turn it slightly so the bevel of the needle is facing up. Puncturing a patient with the bevel down is painful to the patient.
6. Rest the hand with the syringe gently on the desk top. Hold the hand in a position so that when you tilt the point of the needle down slightly, the needle will enter the skin at a 15° angle and about 0.5 centimeters below the point the phlebotomist felt the vein (Fig. 4.8).

Table 4-3   Order of Filling Tubes from a Syringe

1. Blood culture tubes or bottles (sterile procedures)
2. Coagulation "citrate" tube (blue stoppered)
3. Heparin tube (green stoppered)
4. EDTA tube (lavender tube)
5. Oxalate/fluoride tube (gray stoppered)
6. Nonadditive "clot" tubes (red stoppered or gel tubes)

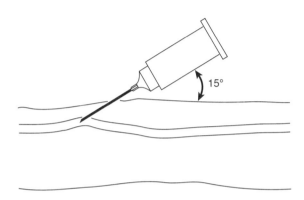

fig 4.8 Proper position of needle entering vein

one hand. The tube will fill itself; do not force the blood into the tube. This technique maintains the proper ratio of blood to anticoagulant. The order of filling the tubes is important as shown in Table 4.3.

Fill sterile collection tubes first to prevent microorganism contamination. The additive tubes are filled before the nonadditive tubes to avoid contamination with microscopic clots. The blood that is last to come out of the syringe was the first blood to go in and has the potential to have started clotting. The empty syringe and needle are then placed into a sharps container without recapping the needle.

Evacuated Tube Specimen Collection

The evacuated tube system is an improvement over the syringe method but maintains many similarities. With the syringe method, as the syringe plunger is pulled, a vacuum is created. The evacuated system has the vacuum already in the tube. Another advantage of the evacuated tube system is that with multiple blood samples, only tubes need to be changed, not syringes.

The similarity of the evacuated tube system is that the holder and needle are held in the same manner as a syringe. A syringe is held in a manner to leave access to pull on the plunger. Access must be left in the evacuated system for one tube to be pulled out and another inserted. The hand that pulled on the plunger of the syringe is the hand that changes tubes with the evacuated system.

The procedure for venipuncture with the evacuated tube system follows the same steps as the syringe method with only slight variation.

EXERCISE 33 — VENIPUNCTURE BY SYRINGE PROCEDURE

Each student uses the anatomical arm to do a syringe venipuncture.

Principle: To obtain venous blood acceptable for laboratory testing as required by a physician.

Specimen: Venous blood collected to be aliquoted into evacuated tubes and/or special collection containers

Equipment:

1. Syringe, vary in size
2. Disposable needle for syringe, 21- or 22-gauge needle
3. Evacuated tube(s) or special collection tube(s)
4. Tourniquet
5. 70 percent isopropyl alcohol swab
6. Gauze or cotton balls
7. Adhesive bandage or tape
8. Sharps container

Procedure:

1. Identify patient. For an in-patient, verify wristband name and hospital number with computer label or requisition information. For an out-patient, ask patient's name and verify with computer label or requisition information.
2. If a fasting specimen is required, ask the patient when he or she last ate.
3. Open the sterile needle and syringe packages, attaching the needle if necessary.
4. Prevent the plunger from sticking by pulling it halfway out and pushing it all the way in one time.
5. Select the proper tube(s) to transfer the blood to after collection.
6. Apply tourniquet.
7. Ask patient to close hand. The patient must not be allowed to pump the hand. Place the patient's arm in a downward position if possible.
8. Select a vein, noting the location and direction of the vein.
9. Clean venipuncture with 70 percent isopropyl alcohol swab.
10. Put on gloves while alcohol is drying. Do not touch venipuncture site.
11. The patient's skin should be drawn taut with the phlebotomist's thumb. The thumb should be 1 to 2 inches below the puncture site.
12. With the bevel up, line up the needle with the vein and perform venipuncture.

EXERCISE **33** VENIPUNCTURE BY SYRINGE PROCEDURE (CONT'D)

13. The vein must not be entered at the exact point the vein was felt. The point the vein was felt is the point where the bevel of the needle must be under the skin. Push the needle into the skin. A sensation of resistance will be followed by easy penetration as the vein is entered. This is known to as feeling the "pop." Once this point is reached, stop and do not move.

14. Take the nondominant hand and pull on the plunger of the syringe. Pull gently and only as fast as the syringe will fill with blood. Pulling too hard or fast will collapse the vein. If the vein does collapse, stop pulling on the plunger and let the vein refill with blood.

15. Pull the plunger back until the desired amount of blood has been obtained.

16. Ask patient to open hand.

17. Release tourniquet.

18. Lightly place gauze square or cotton ball above venipuncture site.

19. Remove needle from arm.

20. Apply pressure to the site for 3 to 5 minutes. The patient may assist if able.

21. Aliquot blood into appropriate tube(s). Puncture stopper of evacuated tube with syringe needle and allow blood to enter tube until flow stops. Mix if any anticoagulant is present. If tube(s) are not evacuated type tubes, remove needle by the needle unwinder on the sharps container or scoop needle cap up one-handed and then unscrew resheathed needle. Blood is then expelled into tube(s) until proper fill.

22. Recheck armband with labels or requisitions.

23. Initial or sign all labels.

24. Label all tubes before leaving the bedside.

25. Apply adhesive bandage.

With multiple draws, the order of drawing the tubes is important. The recommended "order of draw" from a single venipuncture using the evacuated system is as shown in Table 4.4.

Butterfly Collection System

A system that combines the benefits of the syringe system and the evacuated tube system is the butterfly collection system. The butterfly collection system has on one end a 21- or

Table 4–4   Evacuated Tube System Order of Draw

1. Blood culture tubes or bottles (sterile procedures)
2. Nonadditive "clot" tubes (red stoppered or gel tubes)
3. Coagulation "citrate" tube (blue stoppered)
4. Heparin tube (green stoppered)
5. EDTA tube (lavender tube)
6. Oxalate/fluoride tube (gray stoppered)

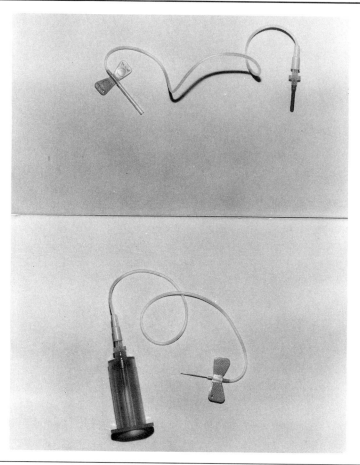

fig 4.9   Butterfly collection set

23-gauge needle with attached plastic wings. Either 6 or 12 inches of tubing leads from the needle. On the other end of this tubing is a hub that can attach to a syringe. A needle covered by a rubber sleeve can also be attached to this tubing. This covered needle screws into an evacuated tube holder (Fig. 4.9).

The butterfly system is for small veins that are difficult to draw with the evacuated tube system and standard evacuated tube system needle. The winged needle of the butterfly system will slide into a small surface vein in the back of the hand, the arm, or the foot. Instead of entering the vein at the usual 15° angle, the winged needle is inserted at approximately a 5° angle and then threaded into the vein. This procedure anchors the needle in the cen-

E X E R C I S E **34**	# VENIPUNCTURE BY EVACUATED TUBE PROCEDURE

Each student uses the anatomical arm to do an evacuated tube venipuncture.

Principle: To obtain venous blood acceptable for laboratory testing as required by a physician.

Specimen: Venous blood collected by evacuated tubes. Volume of blood dependent on size of tube and test requirements.

Equipment:
1. Evacuated tube holder
2. Disposable needle for evacuated system, 20-, 21- or 22-gauge needle
3. Evacuated tube(s) or special collection tube(s)
4. Tourniquet
5. 70 percent isopropyl alcohol swab
6. Gauze or cotton balls
7. Adhesive bandage or tape
8. Sharps container

Procedure:
1. Identify patient. For an inpatient, verify wristband name and hospital number with computer label or requisition information. For an outpatient, ask patient's name and verify with computer label or requisition information.
2. If a fasting specimen is required, ask the patient when he or she last ate.
3. Collect equipment.
4. Break needle seal. Thread the appropriate needle into the holder using the needle sheath as a wrench.
5. Before using, tap all tubes that contain additives to ensure that all the additive is dislodged from the stopper and wall of the tube.
6. Insert the tube into the holder until the needle slightly enters the stopper. Avoid pushing the needle beyond the recessed guideline, because a loss of vacuum may result. If the tube retracts slightly, leave it in the retracted position.
7. Apply tourniquet.
8. Ask patient to close hand. The patient must not be allowed to pump the hand. Place the patient's arm in a downward position if possible.
9. Select a vein, noting the location and direction of the vein.
10. Clean venipuncture site with 70 percent isopropyl alcohol swab.
11. Put on gloves while alcohol is drying. Do not touch venipuncture site.

EXERCISE **34** VENIPUNCTURE BY EVACUATED TUBE PROCEDURE (CONT'D)

12. The patient's skin should be drawn taut with the phlebotomist's thumb. The thumb should be 1 to 2 inches below the puncture site.

13. With the bevel up, line up the needle with the vein and perform venipuncture. Remove your hand from drawing the skin taut. Grasp the flange of the evacuated tube holder and push the tube forward until the butt end of the needle punctures the stopper. You should not change hands while performing the venipuncture. The hand you perform the venipuncture with is the hand that holds the evacuated tube holder. The opposite hand manipulates the tubes.

14. Fill the tube until the vacuum is exhausted and blood ceases to flow into the tube. This will assure the proper ratio of blood to anticoagulant.

15. When the blood flow ceases, remove the tube from the holder. While securely grasping the evacuated tube holder with one hand, use the other hand to change the tubes. The shut-off valve re-covers the point, stopping the flow of blood until the next tube of blood is inserted.

16. Mix immediately after drawing each tube that contains an additive. Gently inverting the tube five to ten times provides adequate mixing without causing hemolysis.

17. Ask patient to open hand.

18. Release tourniquet.

19. Lightly place gauze square or cotton ball above venipuncture site.

20. Remove needle from arm. Be certain last tube drawn has been removed from the holder before removing needle. This will prevent dripping blood out of the tip of the needle.

21. Apply pressure to the site for 3 to 5 minutes. The patient may assist if able.

22. Recheck armband with labels or requisitions.

23. Initial or sign all labels.

24. Label all tubes at the patient's bedside.

25. Apply adhesive bandage.

ter of even a small vein. If the patient moves, the tubing gives flexibility so the needle will stay anchored and not pull out of the vein. The butterfly collection set works well on children that have both small veins and a tendency to move while blood is being collected. The tubing also works as a pressure relief valve: A large evacuated tube or large syringe can be attached to the tubing and the vein will not collapse as would normally occur.

EXERCISE 35 ORDER OF DRAW

The instructor gives five different situations for tubes that need to be drawn from a patient. The students list the tubes in the correct order for filling the tubes.

1. Drawn with an evacuated tube system. Tube colors: green, red, and gray.

2. Drawn with an evacuated tube system. Tube colors: blue, lavender, gel tube, and green.

3. Drawn with a butterfly system. Tube colors: red, blue, lavender, blood culture tubes, and gray.

4. Drawn with a syringe. Tube colors: green, red, and gray.

5. Drawn with a syringe. Tube colors: red, blue, lavender, blood culture tubes, and gray.

The system also gives the adaptability to start drawing blood with a syringe and then finish with the evacuated tube system. A syringe can be used for procedures that require a syringe sample, and then the syringe can be removed and the evacuated tube system attached for multiple tube collection. Even with all of these benefits, the butterfly collection set is not used for all collection. The butterfly collection set is much more expensive than the needle system. This additional expense is unnecessary for the majority of venipunctures.

PATIENT REACTIONS

Patients can have a variety of reactions to having their blood drawn. The phlebotomist must anticipate these reactions and quickly respond with appropriate actions. The most common reaction is pain: The patient will indicate that the venipuncture is painful. Try slightly repositioning the needle and loosening the tourniquet. Loosening the tourniquet often helps because the tourniquet may be pinching the arm and hurting instead of the needle. Avoid deep, probing venipunctures since they go deeper into the skin and get closer to the nerves. If the pain persists, discontinue the venipuncture. Other patient reactions and the phlebotomist's appropriate response are shown in Table 4.5.

THE FAILED VENIPUNCTURE

When a blood sample cannot be obtained, it may be necessary to change the position of the needle. Rotate the needle half a turn. The bevel of the needle may be against the wall of the vein. If the needle has not penetrated the vein far enough, advance it further into the vein. Only advance slightly; a small change is the difference between a failed and a successful venipuncture. If the needle has penetrated too far into the vein, pull back a little.

EXERCISE ▪36▪ VENIPUNCTURE BY BUTTERFLY NEEDLE SYSTEM

Demonstrate the use of a butterfly needle system on an anatomical arm.

Principle: To obtain venous blood acceptable for laboratory testing as required by a physician.

Specimen: Venous blood collected by butterfly needle system. Volume of blood dependent on size of tube and test requirements.

Equipment:
1. Evacuated tube holder
2. Butterfly needle system, 21-, 23-, or 25-gauge needle with or without leur adapter
3. Evacuated tube(s) or special collection tube(s)
4. Tourniquet
5. 70 percent isopropyl alcohol swab
6. Gauze or cotton balls
7. Adhesive bandage or tape
8. Sharps container

Procedure:
1. Identify patient. For an inpatient, verify wristband name and hospital number with computer label or requisition information. For an outpatient, ask patient's name and verify with computer label or requisition information.
2. If a fasting specimen is required, ask the patient when he or she last ate.
3. Collect equipment.
4. Open package of butterfly needle system with leur adapter. Thread the leur needle into the holder.
5. Before use, tap all tubes that contain additives to ensure that all the additive is dislodged from the stopper and wall of the tube.
6. Insert the tube into the holder until the needle slightly enters the stopper. Avoid pushing the needle beyond the recessed guideline, because a loss of vacuum may result. If the tube retracts slightly, leave it in the retracted position.
7. Apply tourniquet.
8. Ask patient to close hand. The patient must not be allowed to pump the hand. Place the patient's arm in a downward position if possible.
9. Select a vein, noting its location and direction.
10. Clean venipuncture site with 70 percent isopropyl alcohol swab.
11. Put on gloves while alcohol is drying. Do not touch venipuncture site.

12. The patient's skin should be drawn taut with the phlebotomist's thumb. The thumb should be 1 to 2 inches below the puncture site.

13. Hold the wings of the butterfly with the bevel up. Line up the needle with the vein and perform venipuncture. Remove your hand from drawing the skin taut. Grasp the flange of the evacuated tube holder and push the tube forward until the butt end of the needle punctures the stopper.

14. Fill the tube until the vacuum is exhausted and blood ceases to flow into the tube. This will assure the proper ratio of blood to anticoagulant. Due to air in the tubing, approximately 0.5 milliliter will be lost when the initial evacuated tube is collected.

15. When the blood flow ceases, remove the tube from the holder. While securely grasping the evacuated tube holder with one hand, use the other hand to change the tubes. The shut-off valve re-covers the point, stopping the flow of blood until the next tube is inserted. Multiple draws require the same order of draw as an evacuated system draw.

16. Immediately after drawing, mix each tube that contains an additive. Gently inverting the tube five to ten times provides adequate mixing without causing hemolysis.

17. Ask patient to open hand.

18. Release tourniquet.

19. Lightly place gauze square or cotton ball above venipuncture site.

20. Remove needle from arm. Be certain last tube drawn has been removed from the holder before removing needle. This will prevent dripping blood out of the tip of the needle.

21. Apply pressure to the site for 3 to 5 minutes. The patient may assist if able.

22. Recheck armband with labels or requisitions.

23. Initial or sign all labels.

24. Label all tubes at the patient's bedside.

25. Apply adhesive bandage.

Variation:

1. Draw with a butterfly system without leur adapter.

2. Instead of threading the leur into the holder in step 4, attach a syringe.

3. Omit step 6.

4. In steps 13, 14, and 15, pull on the syringe instead of pushing the tube into the holder.

5. Aliquot blood from the syringe into appropriate tubes.

Table **4–5** Patient Reactions

Patient Reaction	Phlebotomist Response
Syncope (fainting)	Immediately remove the needle and prevent injury to the patient. Lower the patient's head and arms. Wipe the patient's forehead and back of the neck with a cold compress if necessary. Pass an ammonia inhalant under the patient's nose (the patient will respond by coughing). If the patient still does not respond, a physician must be notified.
Nausea	If a patient becomes nauseated, apply cold compresses to the patient's forehead. Give the patient an emesis basin, and have facial tissues ready if the nausea does not diminish.
Insulin shock/hypoglycemia	The first signs of insulin shock are a cold sweat and pale face, similar to the signs of syncope. The patient becomes weak and shaky, then suddenly becomes mentally confused. This appears as an instant personality change. A physician must be called for the unconscious patient.
Convulsions	The patient becomes unconscious and exhibits violent or mild convulsive motions. Do not try to restrain the patient. Move objects or furniture out of the way to prevent injury to the patient. The patient usually recovers within a few minutes and will be capable of leaving on his/her own after a few minutes of rest.
Cardiac arrest	The patient falls into unconsciousness and has no pulse or respiration. The eyes are dilated, and skin tone is blue or gray. Immediate CPR is necessary to avoid patient death. Only persons certified to do CPR may perform this procedure.

EXERCISE 37 PATIENT REACTIONS

Three pairs of students from the class join in a role play in front of class. One student of each pair plays the phlebotomist; the other is the patient. The patient exhibits reactions, and the phlebotomist reacts to the situation.

Reactions:

Pair 1: Fainting

Pair 2: Nausea

Pair 3: Convulsions

Always "bail out" slowly when the venipuncture has been unsuccessful. The blood will often start coming just as it seems the needle is ready to come out of the skin. The tube being used may not have sufficient vacuum—try another tube before withdrawing.

You can also try stimulating the vein by using the methods listed in Table 4.6.

Probing of the site is not recommended. Probing is painful to the patient and will cause a hematoma. Never attempt a venipuncture more than twice. If a blood sample cannot be obtained in two tries, do a microcollection if possible, or have another person attempt the draw. Notify the patient's physician if two phlebotomists have been unsuccessful and a microcollection is not possible.

INTRAVENOUS AND INDWELLING LINES

Intravenous (IV) lines supply needed fluids and medicines to the patient. When an intravenous solution is being administered into one arm, blood should not be drawn from that arm. Blood drawn from the arm containing the intravenous solution has the potential to contaminate the blood specimen. Intravenous lines are inserted into a vein. The site can be anywhere from the back of the hand to further up the arm. IV sites are generally not placed in the upper area of the arm, but they can be at any site below the upper arm. That makes the upper arm area very tempting to draw blood from because the veins can be felt

Table 4–6 Methods of Vein Stimulation

1. Massage arm in upward motion.
2. Position arm lower than the patient.
3. Reapply the tourniquet.
4. Use a blood pressure cuff in place of the tourniquet.
5. Warm the venipuncture site with a warming device or warm washcloth.

E X E R C I S E 38 VEIN STIMULATION

Three pairs of students from the class join in a role play in front of class. One student of each pair plays the phlebotomist; the other is the patient. The phlebotomist will use one of three methods to stimulate the vein to be more accessible.

Pair 1: Lower patient's arm and retie tourniquet.

Pair 2: Use a blood pressure cuff in place of a tourniquet.

Pair 3: Warm the venipuncture site with a warming device.

in the upper arm and the IV is in the lower part of the arm. Venous blood is flowing up the arm from the hand to the shoulder. The IV solution is flowing in that direction. Any blood drawn in a site above the IV will contain the IV solution. The IV solution will be in a high concentration because it has not had a chance to circulate through the body and distribute through the circulatory system. As a result, the laboratory test results will be high or low, depending on the contents of the IV solution.

To avoid this kind of error, the phlebotomist should look for a blood-drawing site in the opposite arm. Occasionally, an IV will be running in both arms and no site can be found except in the area of the IV. Satisfactory samples can be drawn below the IV by following several precautions. Ask the nurse to shut off the IV for at least 2 minutes before venipuncture. Apply the tourniquet below the IV site. Select a vein other than the one with the IV. Perform the venipuncture. Draw 7 to 10 milliliters of blood, and discard this blood to clear any IV solutions from the arm before test samples are collected. Other alternatives are given in Table 4.7.

A variety of types of cardiovascular (arterial, central venous) or umbilical lines are used on patients. A line is a piece of tubing inserted into the patient's vein or artery. Medications can be administered or blood samples can be taken through this line. Obtaining blood specimens from indwelling lines or catheters can be a source of laboratory test errors if the specimens are not collected properly.

To keep blood from clotting in the line, heparin or saline is used to flush the line. After blood is pulled from the line, heparin or saline is injected into the line until all the blood

---

Table Choices if IV Cannot Be Shut Off

1. Fingerstick blood collection
2. Ankle or foot blood collection
3. Wait until the IV is to be taken out

EXERCISE 39 VENIPUNCTURE SITE

The class is divided into four groups. Each group explains in what locations the blood can be drawn in each of the following situations:

1. IV in the left upper arm

2. IV in the left hand

3. Hematoma on median cubital vein of both arms

4. Mastectomy on right side; IV in left upper arm

is pushed back into the patient. This keeps the line clear until the next blood sample needs to be taken. Any samples first taken from the line will contain a mixture of blood and heparin or saline. At least 7 to 10 milliliters of blood must be discarded to clear all the heparin or saline. After the discard, blood can be drawn as it is drawn from a vein. Not discarding 7 to 10 milliliters of blood will cause erroneous results.

In some situations phlebotomists draw blood from lines, but nurses usually do this type of collection. The same limitations hold for accessing a **cannula**, a type of tubing connector used on kidney transplant or dialysis patients.

Some dialysis patients will have **fistulas**. A fistula is an artificial shunt connection done by a surgical procedure to fuse a vein and an artery. Specimens should be drawn from the opposite arm of a patient with a fistula.

CRITERIA FOR RE-COLLECTION OR REJECTION OF A SPECIMEN

The goal of the phlebotomist is to provide an acceptable specimen for laboratory testing as required by the physician. Certain general criteria must be followed for a specimen to be acceptable. If the criteria are not followed, the specimen must be rejected and re-collected. Table 4.8 gives a list of reasons for rejection of a specimen. This list is not all-inclusive: The type of specimen acceptable and the volume required are determined by the procedure ordered. Re-collection is most often done to recheck results on a patient. When the results from one specimen change significantly from those from a previous specimen, the test will be rechecked. This is done by either retesting the specimen or re-collecting the sample. This will reconfirm the correct patient's blood was drawn and/or the patient's test results did change significantly.

Table **4–8** Reasons for Specimen Rejection

1. A specimen does not have its own label attached to the specimen's primary container.
2. A specimen does not have on its label the test to be performed (CBC, cholesterol, etc.).
3. A label does not have the patient's complete name and hospital number.
4. Specimens are in syringes with needles still attached.
5. Urine specimens do not have the label on the container (where it should be) but on the lid.
6. A specimen is not in its appropriate anticoagulant.
7. Anticoagulated blood collection tubes are not at least 75 percent full. Coagulation blood collection tubes are not at least 90 percent full.
8. Anticoagulated blood specimens not free of clots.
9. Specimens not free of hemolysis and lipemia for certain tests.
10. Blood specimens drawn above an IV site.
11. Urine specimens unrefrigerated for over 2 hours or refrigerated for over 8 hours.
12. Results are not consistent with previous results on the patient. In this case, the specimen must be re-collected.

EXERCISE **40** **REJECTION OF SPECIMEN**

Select five students from the class. Each student is given one situation and is to determine if the specimen is acceptable.

1. The tube of blood is labeled Joe Smith, but an aliquot label on the tube cap has the name Josephine Smith.

2. A blue tube to be used for coagulation testing is half full.

3. A lavender tube to be used for hematology is 80 percent full.

4. The serum of a tube to be tested for potassium is hemolyzed.

5. The hemoglobin of the blood just collected is half of what it was for the same patient on the previous day.

PRIORITIZING SPECIMEN COLLECTION

The phlebotomist is faced with the decision of whose blood to draw first and whose to draw later. Some hospitals allow tests to be ordered with different priorities. The "STAT" test indicates that sample collection is critical to the immediate treatment of the patient. These specimens must be collected before other specimens. The "As Soon As Possible (ASAP)" order priority is sometimes used to indicate that the specimen needs to be collected generally within an hour of the order time. Lesser priorities are "This A.M./P.M." or "Today."

Specimens that must be drawn at a specific time dictate the proper collection time and sequence. STAT specimens should always be collected first. After a STAT specimen is collected, it must not be carried on the phlebotomist's tray while other, lower-priority specimens are collected. The STAT specimen should be taken immediately to the appropriate laboratory.

Certain types of tests determine when the phlebotomist collects the specimen. The blood test for ammonia requires the specimen to be placed on ice and delivered to the laboratory within 20 minutes of collection. If a phlebotomist has several patients from whom to draw blood, one of whom is to have an ammonia test, this patient's blood must be drawn last and then delivered to the laboratory. Each laboratory determines the priority for specimen collection.

ARTERIAL PUNCTURES

Arterial punctures are not for the beginning phlebotomist. Extensive observation and training in the technique should be completed before an arterial puncture is attempted. There is the possibility of serious injury to the patient if arterial samples are not collected correctly. Arterial punctures are used to obtain a specimen for blood gas analysis. This test determines the effectiveness of a patient's ability to absorb gases.

The femoral artery is one of the largest arteries in the body. It is located in the groin and can be palpated and punctured easily due to its size. Pubic hair makes cleansing difficult and can lead to infection. The femoral artery is commonly used for cardiac catheterization and is often reserved only for catheterization-type procedures. Due to many disadvantages of the femoral artery puncture, it is one of the last choices for obtaining arterial blood specimens. Puncture of the femoral artery is generally reserved for physicians.

The brachial artery can be used for arterial punctures but also has several disadvantages. Its location deep within the muscles and connective tissues makes palpating and puncture difficult. Once puncture is completed it is difficult to compress and stop the bleeding. Therefore, hematoma formation is likely.

The preferred puncture site is the radial artery located in the wrist (Fig. 4.10). It is easy to palpate, and the patient is less resistant to a puncture in the wrist. The arm and wrist of

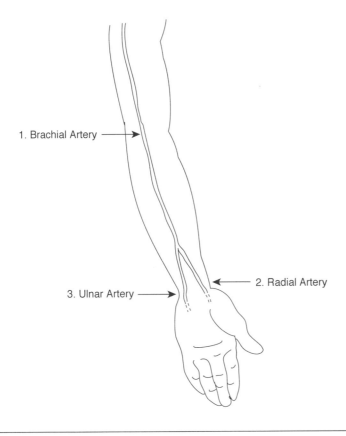

1. Brachial Artery

2. Radial Artery

3. Ulnar Artery

fig 4.10 Arteries in the arm

E X E R C I S E   41   **PULSE**

Have the class divide into pairs. They feel for their own pulse, and then for that of their classmates. They feel for the pulse on the thumb side of the wrist.

EXERCISE **42** **ALLEN TEST**

Have the class divide into pairs. Each pair performs the Allen test on each other.

1. The patient rests the hand with the wrist up.

2. The patient then clenches the fist (Fig. 4.11).

3. Using the middle and index finger of each hand, the phlebotomist presses on the radial and ulnar arteries (Fig. 4.12).

4. While the phlebotomist continues to hold pressure, the patient unclenches the fist (Fig. 4.13).

5. The obstructed flow of blood will cause a blanching of the palm.

6. The palm and fingers should turn pink about 15 seconds after pressure is released only on the ulnar artery (Fig. 4.14). This indicates the ulnar artery is providing circulation to the hand and is refilling the capillary bed.

7. In a negative test the hand will remain blanched, indicating restricted blood flow of the ulnar artery. If the test is a negative, the radial artery of that wrist should not be used and the opposite wrist should be checked.

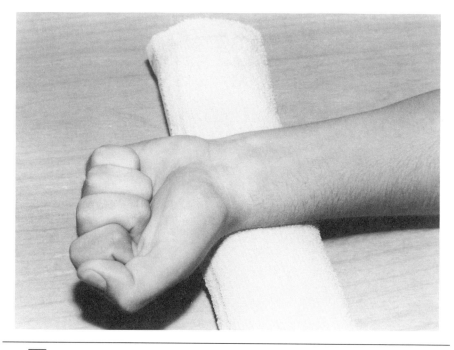

fig **4.11** Allen test: Rest the patient's arm with the wrist up. Have patient clench fist

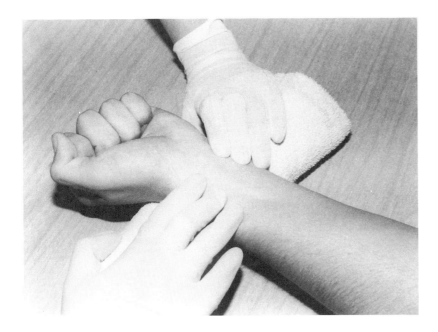

fig 4.12 Apply pressure to the radial and ulnar arteries simultaneously

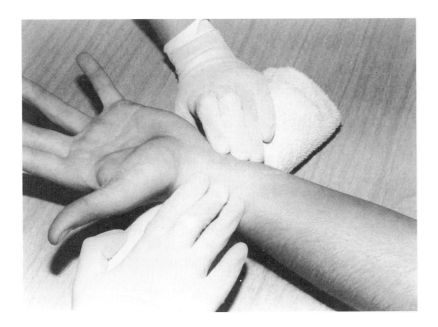

fig 4.13 Have patient unclench fist

the apprehensive patient can be held firmly to prevent movement during sample collection. The artery is also easier to compress after arterial puncture, making hematoma formation less likely. Collateral circulation by the ulnar artery must be checked by use of the Allen test before puncture is made in the radial artery.

The site for the draw of the radial artery is located by feeling with the middle or index finger for a pulsing action; do not use the thumb for palpating. Once the Allen test is per-

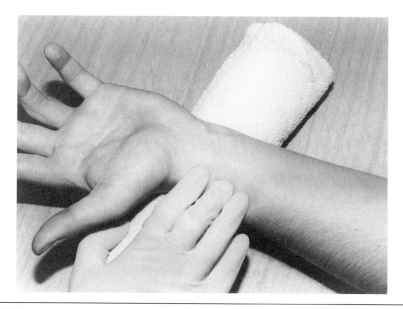

fig 4.14 Release pressure on the ulnar artery. Patient's palm should turn pink

formed and the site is located, the site can be numbed with lidocaine solution. Clean the skin surface with an alcohol prep. Allow the alcohol to air dry. The skin is infiltrated on top of the puncture site with a few drops of anesthetic solution. If the patient is unconscious, or is an adult who is not apprehensive about the arterial puncture, the anesthetic solution may be omitted. A patient who can maintain a stabilized breathing pattern without anesthetic should have the anesthetic step eliminated.

The patient's arm should rest on a table or pillow with the palm facing up and the wrist extended to stretch the arteries and tissues. The artery is then relocated by placing the index or middle finger over the artery to palpate for its size, depth, and direction.

An alternative method for drawing an arterial sample is to use a butterfly needle to puncture the artery. The needle of the butterfly is inserted into the artery using the same method as the syringe technique. Once the butterfly needle is in the artery, the tubing attached to the needle will start filling with blood with a pulsating action. After all the air is forced out of the tubing, a prepared heparin syringe is attached and the arterial blood obtained. The needle is removed from the patient, and the butterfly tubing is detached from the syringe and replaced with a special rubber stopper. Air must not be allowed to enter the syringe. Any air bubbles that enter the syringe must be expelled before the syringe is stoppered.

An alternative to the percutaneous collection of arterial blood samples is to collect them by microcollection through skin puncture. The patient's finger or infant's foot is warmed before the puncture to obtain the maximum arterial blood flow. The capillary bed of the circulatory system is predominantly arterial blood. Blood from the microcollection must be collected in heparinized glass capillary tubes and must not contain air bubbles. Blood is collected directly into the end of the capillary tube without letting it run down the finger or foot. Exposure of the blood to air for as little as 10 to 30 seconds can significantly alter the results of the blood gas test. After collection, one tip of the tube is sealed with clay; a magnetic mixing bar is placed into the opposite end of the tube, and that end is then sealed with clay. The capillary tubes must then be placed on ice immediately. Due to their small size, capillary tubes are more sensitive to temperature variation.

EXERCISE 43 ARTERIAL PUNCTURE

Arterial punctures are done with special arterial-blood-sampling kits that include a preheparinized syringe. Due to the cost of these kits the exercise is done with a 1-milliliter syringe with needle.

1. On an anatomical arm, locate the radial artery.

2. Clean the arterial puncture site with povidone-iodine (Betadine).

3. Paint the skin with the solution, working from the puncture site to the outside in concentric circles, and then let it air dry. The povidone-iodine (Betadine) is not fully effective until it has dried.

4. The artery can no longer be touched except with sterile gloves or fingers that have also been cleaned with povidone-iodine (Betadine).

5. Remove the needle cap from the prepared syringe and hold it as you would a dart.

6. Place your finger over the place in the artery where you want the tip of the needle to be after it has entered the artery.

7. Puncture the skin about 5 to 10 millimeters down the length of the artery (toward the palm) from the point the finger is feeling the pulsating artery.

8. The needle of the syringe should enter the skin at a 45° angle. The bevel of the needle should face the direction of the blood flow (toward the elbow)(Fig. 4.15).

9. This procedure places the bevel of the needle in the center of the artery exactly under the finger that is feeling the pulsating artery.

10. When the artery is punctured, the blood will flow into the syringe. A glass syringe fills faster than a plastic syringe. A plastic syringe sometimes needs a slow gentle pull on the plunger.

11. Once the syringe is filled, the needle must be removed and the syringe opening sealed with a special rubber stopper.

12. The needle can be removed by scooping the needle sheath up with one hand and then unscrewing the needle or by using the slot on a sharps container. Do not try to bend the needle to seal off the syringe. That creates the possibility of accidental puncture.

13. Immediately after the needle is removed, a dry gauze square is placed over the puncture site and pressure applied for a minimum of 5 minutes.

14. Patients on anticoagulant blood thinners will require a longer time to stop the bleeding. Before you leave the patient, check that the artery has not started bleeding again.

EXERCISE **43** **ARTERIAL PUNCTURE (CONT'D)**

15. The specimen must be properly labeled before you leave the patient's room.

16. The specimen is completely immersed in ice water to maintain it at 1° to 5° Celsius. The result obtained from a specimen at 1° to 5° is accurate for 1 to 2 hours, while at room temperature the result is accurate only for 5 to 10 minutes. As soon as the specimen is drawn and labeled, it must be placed in ice water. Waiting until after pressure is held on the patient's arm for 5 minutes will be too long and will invalidate the specimen.

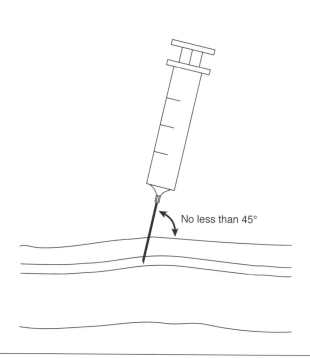

No less than 45°

fig **4.15** Proper position of needle entering artery

SUMMARY

The phlebotomist is the laboratory representative. The patient's response to how well the laboratory performed while the patient was in the hospital will be most influenced by the performance of the phlebotomist. Proper patient and specimen identification is essential to accurate patient testing. The results of sample testing will be wrong if the sample is not accurately identified. The position of the patient is critical to proper blood collection. The position should be comfortable for both the patient and the phlebotomist. Proper positioning of the patient will make the patient feel more at ease, and the phlebotomist will be better able to perform the venipuncture. The three basic techniques to obtain blood by venipuncture are syringe method, evacuated tube method, and butterfly collection system. Patients can have a variety of reactions to having their blood drawn. The phlebotomist must anticipate these reactions and quickly respond with appropriate actions. Arterial samples are reserved for the most experienced phlebotomists due to special precautions that must be taken during collection of the sample.

REVIEW QUESTIONS

Choose the one best answer.

1 The tourniquet should be applied how many inches above the proposed venipuncture site?
   a. 1 to 2 inches
   b. 3 to 4 inches
   c. 4 to 5 inches
   d. 5 to 6 inches

2 Leaving the tourniquet on a patient's arm for an extended length of time before drawing blood may cause:
   a. hemoconcentration
   b. specimen hemolysis
   c. stress
   d. bruising

3 When drawing multiple specimens in evacuated tubes, it is important to fill which of the following color stoppered tubes first?
   a. blue
   b. green
   c. lavender
   d. red

4 The doctor orders tests requiring a blue-top tube for coagulation studies, a lavender-top tube, a red-top tube, and a set of blood cultures. What is the correct order of draw?
   a. red, blue, blood cultures, lavender
   b. blood cultures, blue, lavender, red
   c. blood cultures, red, blue, lavender
   d. blood cultures, green, blue, red

5 As a general rule, you should not stick a patient more than _____ in an attempt to obtain blood.
a. once
b. twice
c. three times
d. four times

6 When you cannot perform a venipuncture successfully after two attempts, you should:
a. try at least two more times
b. notify the patient's physician
c. ask another phlebotomist to try
d. request the test for the next day

7 Why is the first tube discarded when you are drawing from an indwelling arterial line?
a. to remove tissue fluid
b. to wipe away any bacterial contamination
c. to remove heparin/saline contamination
d. to make the blood flow faster

8 Which two arteries are occluded when performing the Allen test?
a. femoral and radial
b. radial and ulnar
c. brachial and ulnar
d. radial and brachial

9 The artery that lies on the thumb side of the wrist is:
a. papliteal
b. radial
c. temporal
d. ulnar

10 Pressure must be applied to the site of an arterial puncture and maintained for at least:
a. 3 minutes
b. 5 minutes
c. 10 minutes
d. 15 minutes

11 In performing an arterial puncture, the artery should be punctured using a:
a. 30° angle of insertion with the bevel of the needle up
b. 30° angle of insertion with the bevel of the needle down
c. 45° angle of insertion with the bevel of the needle up
d. 45° angle of insertion with the bevel of the needle down

12 An arterial puncture site is more likely to bleed than a venipuncture site because of:

a. higher blood pressure in the arteries
b. the lack of specific coagulation factors in arteries
c. lack of elastic tissue in the artery wall
d. the presence of anticoagulant in the arterial syringe

FURTHER ACTIVITIES

Ask the class to describe reactions they have had to having their own blood drawn.

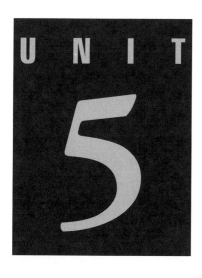

The Challenging Phlebotomy

LEARNING OBJECTIVES

After studying this unit, it is the responsibility of the student to know the following objectives:

- Explain the importance of communication with and reassurance of parents and children.

- Explain the importance of proper holding techniques on children during venipuncture.

- Explain the techniques used in venipuncture in children.

- Describe the composition of skin-puncture blood.

- Describe skin-puncture equipment.

- State the reason that it is important to puncture across the fingerprint line.

- Explain the order of draw for microcollection.

- Explain why hemolysis is more likely in skin-puncture blood.

- Explain what to do after drawing a patient on anticoagulation therapy.

- Explain the best way to handle a resistant patient.

- What the phlebotomist must overcome before a patient in isolation has blood drawn.

GLOSSARY

Capillary Action	Adhesive molecular forces between liquid and solid materials that draw liquid into a narrow-bored capillary tube.
Interstitial Fluid	Fluid located between the cellular components of tissue.

INTRODUCTION

Phlebotomy can be challenging with many patients. Often the veins will not permit a venipuncture. Microcollection of a sample through a skin puncture can provide the phlebotomist with a quality specimen without undue trauma to the patient.

Special phlebotomy skills are needed to obtain blood from special patients. These patients have such problems as continued bleeding or obesity. Phlebotomists also have to work with resistant patients and psychiatric patients. The phlebotomist must follow all safety precautions when collecting a blood sample from a patient in isolation. Knowing special skills and techniques will help the phlebotomist handle all challenging phlebotomy.

VENIPUNCTURE ON CHILDREN

Before drawing blood from a child, the phlebotomist must gain a rapport with the child and the parents. The child will not cooperate with the phlebotomist if the parent is apprehensive and does not show a trust in the phlebotomist. Greet the parent and child calmly and professionally with a soft, understanding voice. Talk to the child, explaining what is going to be done. The child should never be told that it will not hurt but that it will hurt a little bit and that to make it easier they need to hold still.

Limit venipuncture in children younger than 2 years old to superficial veins. Two years old is not a magical age; when more adult-type venipunctures are advisable will vary with each child. Collection of blood from superficial veins generally is most successful with a butterfly collection set and a 23-gauge needle. Once the needle is in the vein, the flexibility of the tubing allows the child to move slightly while the blood is being collected. The butterfly also will have a "flash" of blood in the tubing when the needle enters the vein. Venous collection can be accomplished on children over 2 years old with an evacuated system. Holding the child still is very critical when a syringe or evacuated system is used.

PERFORMING A SKIN PUNCTURE

The skin puncture is the method of choice for children under 1 year old and for adults in whom veins are inaccessible (Table 5.1). As the patient bleeds from the skin puncture, the blood is collected in the appropriate microcollection device. Adult skin punctures are done in the finger; for children under 1 year old the foot is the puncture site of choice. Skin puncture of the earlobe is not recommended. The blood from a skin puncture is from the capillary area of the circulatory system. This blood in the capillary bed is predominantly arterial blood.

EXERCISE 44 HOLDING A CHILD

Have the class divide into pairs. Using large dolls, have each student practice holding the doll while the other student prepares for a venipuncture with an evacuated system.

1. Lay the doll on a table top that will simulate the patient's bed.

2. One student will hold the child down so that the median cubital vein is accessible.

3. Before any attempt is made to hold the child and draw blood, the child is told what is to be done.

4. Tell the child the most important part of having blood drawn is to hold still. Tell the child how you are going to hold him or her so that the child does not feel overwhelmed.

5. For drawing from the child's right arm, the student approaches the child from the left side.

6. The student lays his or her right arm over the child's chest and then holds the child's right shoulder down.

7. This will prevent twisting of the shoulder and raising of the chest during the venipuncture.

8. The student's left arm is placed across the lower part of the body.

9. The left hand holds the child's right wrist to extend the arm.

10. Venipuncture is then performed.

11. After the venipuncture is completed, it is a good idea to have some type of reward. A special "Best Patient" badge or cartoon bandage will make the child feel important and let the parents know you care. The child is a patient who will need some extra minutes of time to make the experience as enjoyable as possible and the job easier for the next phlebotomist.

Any patient who is severely dehydrated or has poor circulation, such as a patient in shock, will not produce an adequate skin-puncture blood sample. A patient who is extremely cold will also not produce adequate blood flow.

A number of different skin-puncture lancets are available. Lancets have been designed to control the depth of puncture. Lancets consist of a lancet blade that is pushed into the skin (Fig. 5.2) or a type of spring-loaded device (Fig. 5.3). The spring-loaded device lies on the surface of the skin, and then the lancet is pushed into the skin or a spring helps make the cut. The rapid puncture and not seeing the blade makes the patient less apprehensive. Avoid using spring lancet devices that are made for glucose monitors. These lancets produce a small, round puncture and produce only 2 to 3 drops of blood. This amount of blood is not sufficient for most laboratory procedures. The devices that produce a small cut cause longer

PREPARING THE PATIENT FOR SKIN PUNCTURE

1. The patient's hand needs to be warmed for skin puncture if there is any coolness in the patient's hand.

2. Warm the hand with a warm washcloth. Warm, wet heat is more efficient than dry heat or a heat pack.

3. The washcloth should be warm to your touch as you carry it to the patient, but not so hot that it burns you. The ideal temperature is 42° Celsius.

4. Wrap the washcloth around the patient's hand for only 3 to 5 minutes. If left on longer, the washcloth will have a cooling effect due to evaporation instead of a warming effect.

5. The heat enlarges the capillaries; blood flow is increased seven times.

6. The site for the collection of a skin puncture in an adult is on the palmar surface of the distal phalanx of the finger (Fig. 5.1). The side or tip of the finger should not be punctured because the tissue is about half as thick as the tissue in the center of the finger.

7. The fingers of choice are the middle finger and the ring finger (second and third fingers).

8. The finger must not be swollen due to the buildup of fluids (edematous). Puncturing an edematous finger will contaminate the sample with the tissue fluid.

9. When puncturing the finger, cut across the fingerprint line. This technique delivers the best possible blood flow and facilitates the formation of drops of blood. If the cut is made between the fingerprint lines, the fingerprints will exert a pressure on the cut and close the cut. Any blood that does flow will follow the lines of the fingerprint, resulting in no droplet formation.

10. Clean the finger with isopropanol (alcohol) and then dry with a sterile gauze or allow to air dry thoroughly before any puncture.

11. Alcohol that is not dry contaminates the blood sample, and the sample will become hemolyzed. Do not use povidone iodine (Betadine) to clean and disinfect the puncture site. Even if the Betadine has been allowed to dry, it will cause an elevated potassium, phosphorous, or uric acid test result.

Table 5-1 Reasons for Skin Puncture

1. Severely burned patients
2. Oncology patients for whom the veins are reserved for therapeutic purposes.
3. Obese patients in whom veins are too deep to locate.
4. Geriatric patients or other patients in whom veins are not accessible or are very fragile.
5. Patients performing tests on themselves (home glucose monitoring).
6. Special procedures that require capillary blood (malarial smears or Unopette platelets).
7. Children who have inaccessible veins.
8. When the amount of blood taken from the patient must be limited, for example, premature babies

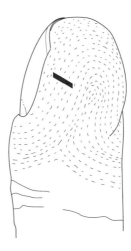

fig 5.1 Puncture site on finger

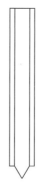

fig 5.2 Lancet

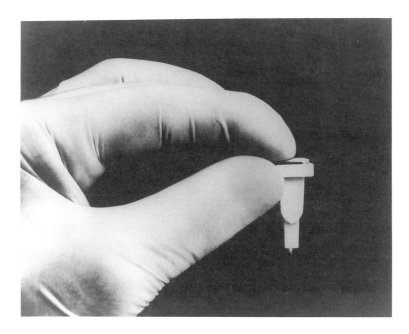

fig 5.3 Example of spring-loaded lancet (courtesy of Becton Dickinson VACUTAINER Systems)

bleeding and produce a sufficient amount of blood. The depth of the cut for adults varies depending on the device used. It is better to puncture deeply enough the first time, so that all the blood can be obtained, rather than to need to puncture more than once.

Plan for the drop of blood from the puncture. As the patient's hand is held, the underside of the finger is the side to be punctured. After the puncture, the blood will drip downward, and gravity will help the blood flow into the collector. Before the blood sample is collected, the first drop of blood will need to be wiped away. As the finger is punctured, tissue cells are damaged and **interstitial fluid** is released into the first drop. The subsequent drops are blood because it is flowing due to the arterial pressure.

The devices used for collecting, processing, and transporting microcollections vary depending on the laboratory test being performed. Disposable capillary micropipettes are devices much like a glass soda straw (Fig. 5.4). The blood draws up into the tube because of **capillary action**. Capillary action is the adhesive molecular force between liquid and solid materials that draws liquid into narrow-bored capillary tubes.

The process of collecting and transporting blood samples has been simplified with the use of microcollection devices. These devices offer a method for filling, measuring, color coding for proper anticoagulant, stoppering, centrifugation, and storage in one tube. As the drop of blood forms, it is touched by the collection cap, which consists of a scoop or tubing device. A tube holds approximately 600 microliters of blood. Tubes can be purchased in a variety brands, such as Microtainer, or Microvette (Fig. 5.5).

If the puncture is adequate, 0.5 milliliters of blood can be collected from a single puncture. A drop of blood will form at the puncture site. As the drop of blood forms, the tip of the microcollection device is touched to the drop of blood. Blood flow can be further enhanced by gently applying continuous pressure to the surrounding tissue. Rapid milking of the finger will not enhance the blood flow. Excess pressure will cause hemolysis or contamination of the specimen with tissue fluid.

The microcollection device is held so the drops of blood can flow into its tip and then down the walls of the device. If blood lodges in the tip of the device, tapping the device on

EXERCISE 46 FINGERSTICK SKIN PUNCTURE

The class is divided into pairs and does a fingerstick blood collection on each other.

Principle: To obtain capillary blood acceptable for laboratory testing as requested by a physician.

Specimen: Capillary blood volume dependent on the test(s).

Equipment

1. Disposable sterile lancet
2. Sterile gauze squares
3. Alcohol swabs
4. Gloves
5. Collection containers, as required by test(s):
   a. Capillary tubes
   b. Diluting fluids
   c. Calibrated pipettes
   d. Microcollection containers

Procedure

1. Apply gloves before any patient contact.
2. Identify patient. For an inpatient, verify wristband name and hospital number with computer label or requisition information. For an outpatient, ask name and verify with computer label or requisition information.
3. Verify collection orders.
4. Choose a finger that is not cold or edematous for the puncture site.
5. If all fingers are cold, warm the hand 3 minutes with a warm washcloth.
6. Select the appropriate containers for blood collection.
7. An ambulatory patient should be seated in a standard phlebotomy chair with armboard. A supine (lying down) patient should have the arm lowered to a position slightly lower than the breastbone.
8. Gently massage the finger using a milking action to increase blood flow potential (Fig. 5.6).
9. Clean the puncture site with alcohol and let the area dry (Fig. 5.7).
10. Puncture the skin with the disposable lancet (Fig. 5.8).
11. Wipe away the first drop of blood with a sterile dry gauze (Fig. 5.9).
12. Collect the specimen in the chosen container. Touch only the tip of the collection tube to the drop of blood. Blood flow is encouraged if the puncture site is held at a downward angle and a gentle pressure applied to the finger (Fig. 5.10).

E X E R C I S E | **46** | **FINGERSTICK SKIN PUNCTURE (CONT'D)**

13. Seal the specimen container.

14. Apply a bandage to the puncture site. A bandage should be omitted on infants and small children because they may swallow the bandage and choke.

15. Label the collection containers

16. If insufficient sample has been obtained, the puncture may be repeated at a different site. A new sterile lancet and new collection containers must be used.

17. Remove gloves and wash hands before going to the next patient.

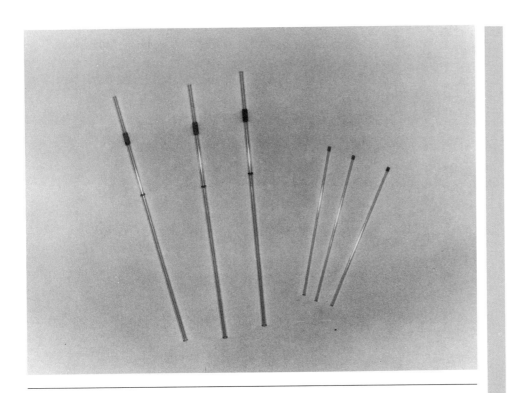

fig **5.4** Calibrated micropipettes and microhematocrit tubes

a hard surface will facilitate the blood flow. The tube should be rotated after every drop so that the blood entering the tube will contact the anticoagulant coating the sides. Anticoagulant specimens should be mixed by inverting 8 to 10 times.

For some microcollections, the phlebotomist will be required to set up the test at the patient's bedside by collecting the sample and then making dilutions of the sample. A micropipette and dilution system are used to make this task easier (Fig. 5.11). The brand

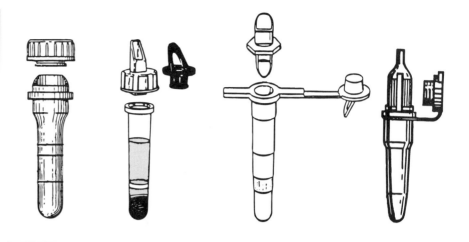

fig 5.5 Microcollection devices (reproduced with permission from H14-A2 *Devices for Collection of Skin Puncture Blood Specimens,* 2nd ed. Approved Guideline. NCCLS, 771 E. Lancaster Avenue, Villanova, PA 19085)

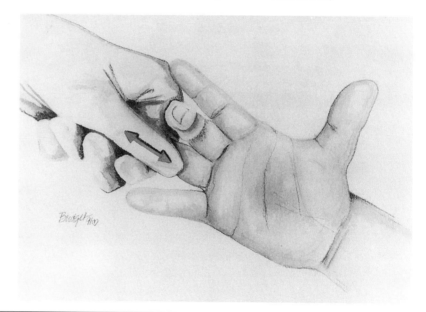

fig 5.6 The ambulatory patient should be seated in a standard phlebotomy chair with an arm board. This position improves fingertip blood pressure and perfusion. A supine patient should have the arm lowered to a position slightly below the breastbone. When the patient is in this position, gently massage the entire length of the finger using a milking action. This increases the temperature of the finger and improves perfusion. (Reprinted with permission from International Technidyne Corporation.)

name for this type of system is the Unopette system, manufactured by Becton Dickinson. The system consists of a plastic reservoir that contains a premeasured amount of reagent, a capillary pipette that fits into a plastic holder, and a pipette shield. The reservoir is punctured to open access to the reagent. Blood is drawn into the pipette. The filled pipette is rinsed to dilute the blood in the reagent. These devices are used for such tests as platelet counts, hemoglobin determinations, and WBC and RBC counts.

The last microcollection method we discuss is blood collection on filter paper for neona-

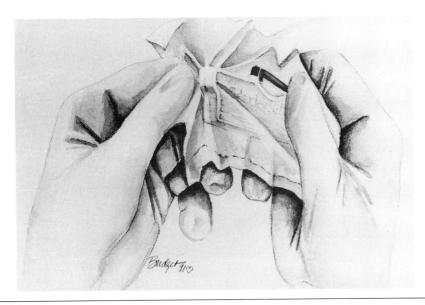

fig 5.7 Clean the incision site and let it air dry. Remove the lancet device from its plastic packet, taking care not to touch or contaminate the blade-slot surface or contoured edge. (Reprinted with permission from International Technidyne Corporation.)

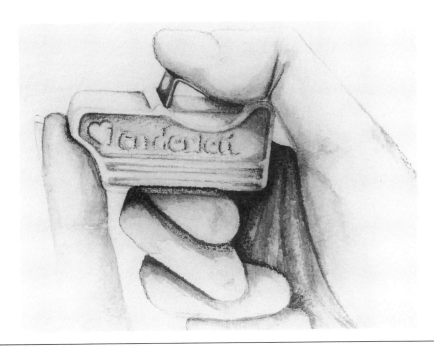

fig 5.8 Again gently massage the lower portion of the finger while avoiding the fingertip incision site. Then firmly grasp the lower portion of the finger to restrict return circulation. Firmly position the lancet device on the finger and depress the trigger. (Reprinted with permission from International Technidyne Corporation.)

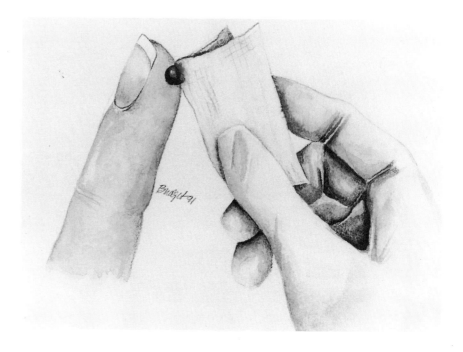

fig 5.9 After triggering, immediately remove the instrument from the patient's finger. Using a sterile gauze pad, gently wipe the first droplet of blood. Gentle, continuous pressure to the finger assures a good blood flow. (Reprinted with permission from International Technidyne Corporation.)

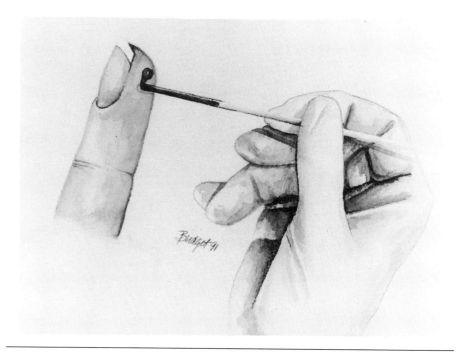

fig 5.10 Taking care not to make direct contact between the wound and the collection container or capillary tube, fill to the desired specimen volume. Following collection, gently press a dry gauze pad to the incision. (Reprinted with permission from International Technidyne Corporation.)

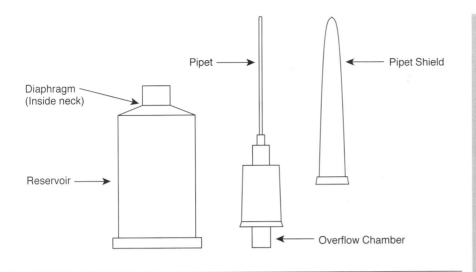

fig 5.11 Unopette (reproduced with permission from H14-A2 *Devices for Collection of Skin Puncture Blood Specimens,* 2nd ed. Approved Guideline. NCCLS, 771 E. Lancaster Avenue, Villanova, PA 19085)

tal screening programs (Fig. 5.12). These programs screen newborns for genetic defects. The newborn is punctured in the heel, and the blood is dropped onto a filter paper card. The blood is allowed to dry, and the blood-saturated filter paper is tested. Infants can be tested in this manner for phenylketonuria, galactosemia, hypothyroidism, homocystinuria, maple sugar urine disease, and sickle cell disease/hemoglobinopathies. With early identification of these diseases, treatment will lessen the disorder and often completely prevent it.

OBTAINING A BLOOD SAMPLE FROM A BABY

To obtain a blood microcollection sample on a child under 1 year old, the phlebotomist follows many of the same procedures as a fingerstick sample; the main difference is the puncture site. For infants and young children the heel is the puncture site of choice. If an infant's heel is to be punctured, the site should be on the plantar surface medial to a line drawn posteriorly from the middle of the great toe to the heel, or lateral to a line drawn posteriorly from between the fourth and fifth toes to the heel (Fig. 5.13). In almost all infants the bones, arteries, and nerves are not near these areas. On the inside (big toe side) of the heel, a posterior tibial artery is near the curvature of the heel. The outside of the heel (little toe side) is the primary area of choice in heel puncture. The inside (big toe side) of the heel can be used as long as puncture depth is controlled. The puncture should not be done in a previous puncture site due to the possibility of infection. Do not do punctures in the central arch area of the foot. Puncture in this area may result in damage to nerves, tendons, and cartilage and offers no advantage to a heel puncture.

The optimal depth of skin puncture from which an adequate blood sample can be obtained without injury to the infant is 2.4 millimeters. The capillary bed of the infant is 0.35 to 1.6 millimeters beneath the skin surface. A puncture of the plantar surface of the heel to a depth of 2.4 millimeters will puncture the major capillary beds and not injure the bone or nerves of the heel. Numerous devices are commercially available that meet the requirement of a puncture of 2.4 millimeters deep or less.

Puncture of an infant's fingers should be avoided. The distance to the bones and main

EXERCISE 47 UNOPETTE PROCEDURE

1. *Puncture diaphragm:* Using the protective shield on the capillary pipette, puncture the diaphragm of the reservoir as follows:
   a. Place the reservoir on a flat surface. Grasping the reservoir in one hand, take pipette assembly in the other hand and push tip of pipette shield firmly through diaphragm in neck of reservoir, then remove.
   b. Remove shield from pipette assembly with a twist.
   c. Gloves must be worn before fingerstick and during the remaining procedure.

2. *Add sample:* After fingerstick of the patient and wiping away the first drop of blood, the capillary must be filled with whole blood and transferred to the reservoir as follows:
   a. Holding the pipette almost horizontally, touch tip of pipette to the blood from the finger puncture. Pipette will fill by capillary action. Filling is complete and will stop automatically when blood reaches end of capillary bore in neck of pipette.
   b. Wipe excess blood from outside of capillary pipette, making certain that no sample is removed from capillary bore.
   c. Squeeze reservoir slightly to force out some air. Do not expel any liquid. Maintain pressure on reservoir.
   d. Cover opening of overflow chamber with index finger and seat pipette securely in reservoir neck.
   e. Release pressure on reservoir. Then remove finger from pipette opening. Negative pressure will draw blood into diluent.
   f. Squeeze reservoir gently two or three times to rinse capillary bore, forcing diluent into, but not out of, overflow chamber. Pressure is released each time to return the mixture to the reservoir.
   g. Place index finger over upper opening and gently invert five to six times to mix blood thoroughly with diluent.
   h. The specimen is then labeled and taken to the laboratory.

3. *Sources of error:*
   a. Squeezing the reservoir and spilling some of the liquid will give an inaccurate result.
   b. While wiping the outside of the capillary pipette, any blood drawn out of the tube will lower the expected results.
   c. Not wiping the blood from the outside of the capillary pipette will increase the expected results.
   d. Bubbles in the capillary pipette or incomplete filling of the capillary pipette will lower the expected results.
   e. Using a reservoir that has a punctured diaphragm will give inaccurate results.

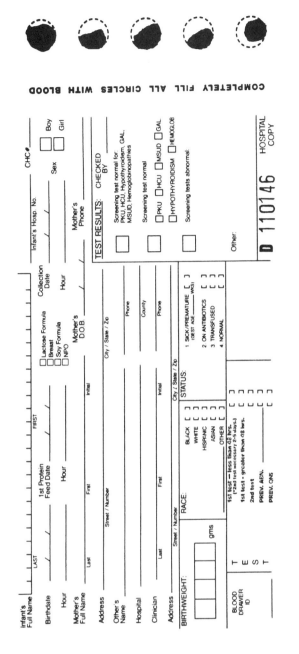

fig 5.12 Newborn screen filter paper collection

nerves of the infant's fingers is 1.2 to 2.2 millimeters. Most lancets are longer than this, and puncture of the infant's finger would damage the bone or nerves, with subsequent infection or permanent physical damage. The infant's finger will also not produce an adequate blood specimen.

An infant's excessive crying can result in elevated leukocyte counts. The leukocyte count will not return to normal for up to 60 minutes. An infant that has had a procedure completed, such as circumcision, will need at least 60 minutes after crying for a blood sample not to have falsely elevated values.

Several precautions must be observed to produce the most accurate specimen. Hemolysis is the greatest concern with microcollection samples (Table 5.2).

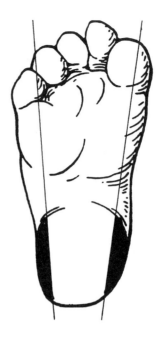

fig 5.13 Infant heel: The darkened areas illustrate the acceptable areas for puncture. The little toe side is the primary area of choice

Table 5-2 Causes of Hemolysis

1. The alcohol used to clean the skin was not allowed to dry.
2. The finger or heel was squeezed to produce a greater blood flow.
3. Newborn infants have increased fragility of red blood cells and a high volume of red blood cells. These factors result in a higher amount of hemolysis.
4. Instead of the blood being allowed to flow into the microcollection container, the blood was scrapped off the skin surface.

Hemolysis, as measured by the concentration of free hemoglobin in the serum or plasma of the blood, may not be readily apparent. This is particularly so in the case of those newborns with elevated bilirubins. The yellow color of the serum may mask hemolysis.

Producing a specimen without clots is also a challenge in microcollection. The body turns on its defenses to clot the blood at the puncture site and stop the bleeding as soon as the skin is punctured. These defenses create problems when a whole-blood sample is needed. If an EDTA specimen is required, the EDTA specimen is drawn first to obtain an adequate volume before the blood starts to clot. Any other additive specimens are collected next, and clotted specimens are collected last. If the blood has started to produce microscopic clots while filling the last tube, there is not a problem because the blood is going to be allowed to clot in the tube.

EXERCISE **48** HEELSTICK SKIN PUNCTURE

Principle: To obtain capillary blood acceptable for laboratory testing as requested by a physician.

Specimen: Capillary blood volume dependent on the test(s).

Equipment

1. Disposable sterile lancet with a blade 2.4 millimeters long or less
2. Sterile gauze squares
3. Alcohol swabs
4. Gloves
5. Collection containers, as required by test(s)
   a. Capillary tubes
   b. Diluting fluids
   c. Calibrated pipettes
   d. Microcollection containers

Procedure

1. Apply gloves before contact with any patient.
2. Identify patient. For an inpatient, verify wristband name and hospital number with computer label or requisition information. For an outpatient, ask name from the person bringing the infant in for testing and verify with computer label or requisition information.
3. Verify collection orders.
4. Choose the heel that is not cold or edematous for the puncture site.
5. Warm the foot for 3 minutes with a warm washcloth or heel warmer.
6. Select the appropriate containers for blood collection.
7. With the baby lying down, clean the puncture site with alcohol and let the area dry (Fig. 5.14).
8. Remove the lancet device from the package, taking care not to touch the blade slot to any nonsterile surface (Figs. 5.15 and 5.16).
9. Raise the baby's heel above heart level, and carefully select a safe incision site. Place the blade slot of the device flush against the heel so that its center point is vertically aligned with the desired incision site. Depress the trigger. Remove the instrument from the baby's heel (Fig. 5.17).
9. Wipe away the first drop of blood with a sterile dry gauze (Fig. 5.18).
10. Collect the specimen in the chosen container. Touch only the tip of the collection tube to the drop of blood. Blood flow is encouraged if the puncture site is held at a downward angle and a gentle pressure is applied to the foot. Following collection, place a dry gauze pad on the incision (Fig. 5.19).

EXERCISE **48** HEELSTICK SKIN PUNCTURE
(CONT'D)

11. Apply a bandage to the puncture site.

12. Label the collection containers.

13. If insufficient sample has been obtained, the puncture may be repeated at a different site. A new sterile lancet must be used and steps 2 to 12 must be repeated.

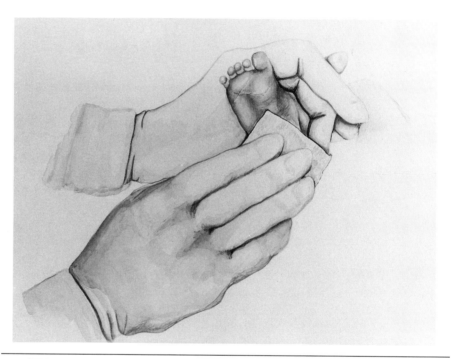

fig **5.14** The ideal posture for this procedure is with the baby in a supine position with the knee at the open end of the bassinet. Clean the incision area of the heel with an antiseptic swab. Allow the heel to air dry. Do not touch the incision site or allow the heel to come in contact with any nonsterile item or surface. (Reprinted with permission from International Technidyne Corporation.)

SPECIAL PATIENTS

The Patient on Anticoagulation Therapy

The patient on anticoagulation therapy presents a special challenge to the phlebotomist. The patient who has been on anticoagulants to "thin the blood" is susceptible to continued bleeding and hematomas. The tendency toward continued bleeding should be treated after venipuncture by holding pressure on the site for at least 5 minutes.

A patient who immediately bleeds through the gauze square should have several layers

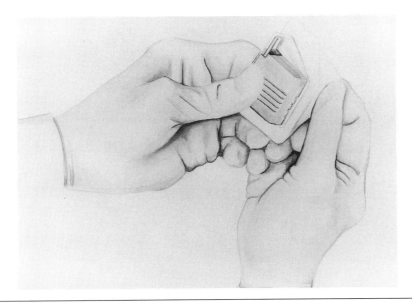

fig 5.15 Remove the lancet device from the package, taking care not to rest the blade slot on any nonsterile surface. (Reprinted with permission from International Technidyne Corporation.)

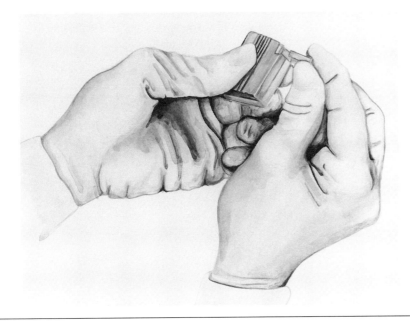

fig 5.16 Remove the safety clip. Do not push on the trigger or touch the blade slot. (Reprinted with permission from International Technidyne Corporation.)

of gauze placed over the site and the arm wrapped with an elastic bandage. The nurse must be told of excessive bleeding to monitor the patient further.

The Resistant Patient

The resistant patient can be one who is aware of what she or he is doing and simply does not want blood drawn. The resistant patient can also be one who is semiconscious

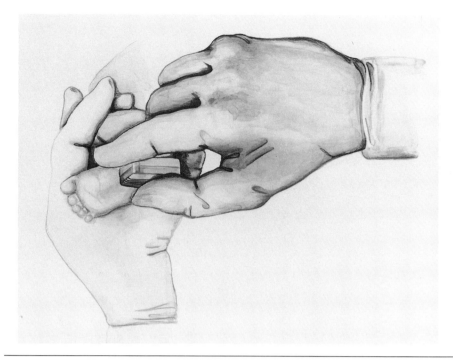

fig 5.17 Raise the foot above the baby's heart level and carefully select a safe incision site. Place the blade-slot surface of the device flush against the heel so its center point is vertically aligned with the desired incision site. Depress the trigger. Remove the instrument from the infant's heel. (Reprinted with permission from International Technidyne Corporation.)

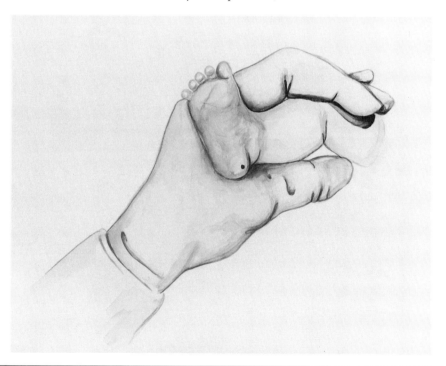

fig 5.18 Using a dry sterile gauze pad, gently wipe the first droplet of blood. (Reprinted with permission from International Technidyne Corporation.)

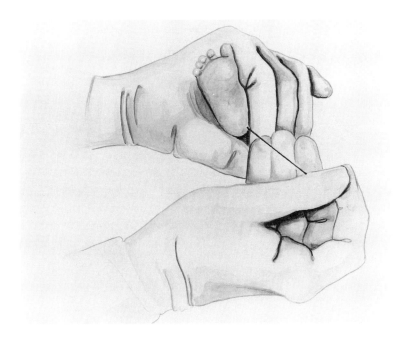

fig `5.19` Taking care not to make direct contact with the collection container or capillary tube, fill to the desired specimen volume. Following collection, gently press a dry gauze pad to the incision. (Reprinted with permission from International Technidyne Corporation.)

or comatose and is unaware of his or her actions. The patient who is aware of his or her actions does have the right to refuse to have blood drawn. In this case, the doctor must be notified to convince the patient that the blood work is essential to the patient's recovery.

The patient who is unaware of her or his actions can have blood drawn, but the phlebotomist will need assistance in holding the patient still. Have the patient's nurse present so it can be documented in the patient's chart that the patient was held to draw the requested blood sample but not injured in the process.

The Psychiatric Patient

The psychiatric patient often does not understand what is being done. When blood is drawn in a psychiatric area, the patient's nurse will need to be informed that blood is to be drawn. The nurse will often accompany the phlebotomist to the patient's room to help explain the procedure to the patient or to help hold the patient. Some psychiatric patients are suicidal. You should be watchful of your equipment to prevent the patient's taking items that could be used to harm the patient or someone else.

The Obese Patient

The obese patient often has veins that are difficult to feel due to the layers of tissue that must be felt through to palpate a vein. The tourniquet will have to be rather tight to exert pressure deep enough to slow the flow of venous blood. Before a venipuncture is attempted, follow the course of the vein. Obese patients have localized tissue globules under their skin that resemble veins when first felt, but these "veins" do not continue and will not result in blood return. The median cubital vein is usually the most prominent vein to feel. If the median cubital vein cannot be found, the veins in the hand and wrist will be more readily accessible. If no vein can be found, consider the fingerstick as an alternative.

The Patient in Isolation

No matter how many patients have blood drawn a day, the phlebotomist still is often hesitant to go into an isolation room to be subjected to an infection. This fear will decrease with experience and knowledge of the isolation procedures used to protect the associate and the patient (See Unit 2, Safety in Phlebotomy). The patient in isolation is also a challenge because of the extra protection the phlebotomist must wear while drawing blood. This extra protection makes the job slower but safer. The protection is for the benefit of both the phlebotomist and the patient.

The Patient with Damaged or Collapsing Veins

Obtaining a blood sample from a patient can be challenging as a result of the patient's veins. The veins can be damaged and healed improperly. This is usually the result of the patient having been burned, scars on the veins through drug abuse or accidents, or surgical procedures in the areas of the veins. The damage results in the veins being inaccessible because the scar tissue is too thick or the vein no longer carries blood.

A collapsing vein is a vein that is weak, and the vacuum of the syringe or evacuated tube "sucks" the walls of the vein together so no blood can flow. The vein refills the instant the vacuum is discontinued. An evacuated system can be used to draw from a collapsing vein, but only small tubes can be used. The larger the evacuated tube, the more vacuum there is in the tube. If a 15-milliliter tube collapses the vein, draw five 3-milliliter tubes instead to obtain the same volume.

EXERCISE **49** SPECIAL PATIENTS

Divide the class into six groups. Each group explains the steps they would take in drawing each type of special patient:

1. The patient on anticoagulation therapy

2. The resistant patient

3. The psychiatric patient

4. The obese patient

5. The patient in isolation

6. The patient with damaged or collapsing veins

A syringe is the best method to use to obtain blood from a collapsing vein. The syringe plunger is pulled gently a small pull at a time. The timing between pulls allows the vein to refill. During each pull on the syringe, a small amount of blood will enter the syringe. Do not work so slowly that the blood starts to clot in the syringe.

SUMMARY

The challenging phlebotomy is due to the patient and not the ability of the phlebotomist. Many patients do not have the large veins that are easy to access. These veins can be small or can continue to collapse when venipuncture is attempted. These patients consist of children and adults. Often the best way to obtain blood is through a skin puncture. With the skin puncture, the sample is smaller and the devices used are different than for a venipuncture. The phlebotomist also must learn to use special techniques and skills to work with special patients such as those on anticoagulation therapy, resistant, psychiatric, obese, or those in isolation.

REVIEW QUESTIONS

Choose the one best answer.

1 The depth of the cut made by a lancet for a heel puncture must be no deeper than:
   a. 3 millimeters
   b. 2.8 millimeters
   c. 2.4 millimeters
   d. 1.5 millimeters

2 The safe area for heel punctures in an infant is:
   a. the arch of the foot
   b. the curvature of the heel
   c. the most medial or lateral portion of the plantar surface
   d. through previous puncture sites

3 Why must the first drop of blood from a capillary puncture be wiped away?
   a. to remove tissue fluid contamination
   b. to wipe away any bacterial contamination
   c. to remove heparin contamination
   d. to make the blood flow faster

4 Warming the skin puncture site:
   a. increases sevenfold the blood flow through the arterioles and capillaries
   b. results in hemolysis of the blood sample
   c. should be performed with a hot towel (60° Celsius)
   d. should not be done routinely because it could alter the chemical values in the blood

5 Blood obtained by skin puncture is more likely to be contaminated by:
a. hemoconcentration
b. glycolysis
c. hemotoma
d. hemolysis

6 If blood is drawn too quickly from a small vein, the vein will have a tendency to:
a. bruise
b. collapse
c. disintegrate
d. roll

7 The following items are essential information for specimen labeling:
a. the patient's complete name, the identification number, date and time the specimen was obtained, and the name of the physician
b. the patient's complete name, the identification number, and date and time the specimen was obtained
c. the patient's complete name and the identification number
d. the patient's complete name and the date and time the specimen was obtained

8 A conscious patient does not have an identification armband. The name and room number on the door agree with that on the request. What should the phlebotomist do?
a. Ask the patient for verbal verification of his or her name.
b. Draw the patient's blood and take the specimen to the lab.
c. Do not draw the patient's blood until an armband has been applied.
d. Draw the patient's blood and then ask the nurse to identify the patient.

9 A phlebotomist is requested to draw blood from an unconscious patient. The room number and the name on the door agree with the request form and the patient identification armband. What else should be done to ensure patient identification?
a. Attempt to awaken the patient for verbal verification of identification.
b. Attempt to find the patient's name on some other item in the room.
c. Nothing else is necessary.
d. Obtain verification from a relative or a nurse as to the patient's identification.

10 An unconscious, unidentified man is admitted to an emergency trauma center. What is the system of choice to ensure patient identification?
a. Assign a name to the patient, such as John Doe, and use that name for identification.
b. Assign a number to the patient until the patient can be identified.
c. Wait to process any samples until the patient can be identified.
d. Use a three-part identification system that utilizes a temporary armband and labels for specimens and blood to be transfused.

FURTHER ACTIVITIES

Give the class a demonstration of the different types of lancets available and the different types of microcollection devices available. Discuss the advantages and disadvantages of each device.

Using colored water and capillary pipettes, experiment with the capillary action of the pipettes.

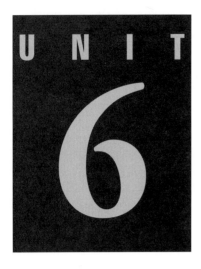

Specimen Considerations and Special Procedures

LEARNING OBJECTIVES

After studying this unit, it is the responsibility of the student to know the following objectives:

- Explain the importance of a fasting specimen.

- Explain the importance of a timed specimen.

- Explain the importance of specimen drawing in monitoring therapy.

- Describe how a STAT specimen should be handled.

- Describe the proper procedure for making a blood smear.

- List the characteristics of a good slide.

- Explain the procedure of a glucose tolerance test and the two variations of how the glucose drink is administered.

- Describe the correct procedure for a bleeding time test.

- Explain why a bleeding time test is performed.

- Explain the importance of proper skin antisepsis in blood culture collection.

- List at least four factors that affect laboratory test values.

- Describe the specimen collection and handling procedures for urinalysis specimens.

GLOSSARY

Diurnal	Daily occurrence at a particular time of day.
Fasting	Having had nothing to eat for at least 12 hours.
NPO	Nothing by mouth
Postprandial	After a meal.
Septicemia	A condition in which microorganisms (mainly bacteria) are circulating and multiplying in the patient's blood

INTRODUCTION

The phlebotomist plays an integral role in a patient's health care. The impact of the phlebotomist's knowledge is critical to special procedures. The phlebotomist needs to inquire whether the patient has eaten or when was the last time the patient ate. To provide the most accurate results, the phlebotomist also needs to determine from the nurse or physician the patient's timing for receiving drug therapy so that the venipuncture can be timed appropriately.

When the phlebotomist is on the nursing units and away from the laboratory, the phlebotomist must be independent and knowledgeable enough to handle different situations. The situation may vary, from organizing a series of emergency requests to determining an acceptable blood smear to take to the laboratory.

FASTING SPECIMENS

Some tests must be collected while the patient is **fasting**. A fasting specimen is collected from a patient in the morning, before the patient has had breakfast and before any activities. In addition to fasting to ensure accurate test results, some tests require diet restrictions. No alcohol for a number of hours before the test, or a limit on certain foods are some of the restrictions. Some foods or drinks mask the results the physician is looking for. The patient's nurse should be informed that you have just drawn blood from a patient for fasting blood work so that the nurse can release the restrictions.

TIMED SPECIMENS

Some specimens must be drawn at timed intervals because of medication and/or biological rhythms. These specimens should be collected at the precise time intervals required. Tests that exhibit a **diurnal** effect are those for serum iron, corticosteriods, and other hormones. Such specimens are often drawn 12 hours apart in the early morning and afternoon.

Levels for certain therapeutic drugs are measured to determine how effective the drug is in the patient. Since patients vary in how they respond to a therapeutic drug, each patient must be tested. The patient is tested before the drug is given (prespecimen) and then after the drug has been administered (postspecimen).

The prespecimen is drawn when the therapeutic drug is at the lowest level in the patient; this level is the trough level. The specimen for the trough level is usually drawn 5 minutes before the drug is administered. The drug is administered either through an IV over a timed period or intermuscularly. The drug will vary in the amount of time it is administered if given through an IV. Usually the drug is administered over 30 minutes to 1 hour. Once the drug is administered, the postspecimen is collected. The postspecimen, drawn when the drug is at its highest level in the body, is also called the peak specimen. In general, the postspecimen is drawn 5 minutes after infusion.

The critical step for the phlebotomist is documenting the accurate time of collection. The phlebotomist must check the drug has not yet been given at the time of prespecimen collection.

STAT SPECIMENS

STAT specimens must have the phlebotomist's immediate attention. A STAT order is critical; not obtaining and processing it immediately could lead to the death of the patient. There is a large variability in the criticalness of the STAT. Some hospitals have instituted different levels of the STAT test, or a middle-of-the-road priority such as "As Soon As Possible" (ASAP).

SPECIAL COLLECTION TECHNIQUES

Some tests require special collection techniques for the accuracy of the procedure.

Alcohol

When blood is drawn for alcohol testing, a disinfectant solution other than alcohol must be used. Swabbing the phlebotomy site with alcohol, even when allowed to dry, will contaminate the blood specimen and falsely raise the alcohol level of the patient. Solutions such as zephrin chloride, soap, or hydrogen peroxide are acceptable. Do not use Betadine or iodine swabs because these contain alcohol. Care must also be taken with these specimens because the results are often needed for legal reasons.

Legal Specimens

For specimens obtained for legal reasons, the results of which may be used in a court case, a special chain-of-custody procedure should be followed. The chain-of-custody procedure dictates that each person handling the specimen signs a form. The form indicates from whom each signer received the specimen, to whom it was given, and the length of time each signer had the specimen. The specimen is also transported in a locked box to prevent the possibility of switching or tampering with the specimen. This chain of custody guarantees to the court the integrity of the specimen.

Heavy Metals

A special procedure is to be followed when the blood is to be tested for heavy metals such as arsenic or lead. These are sometimes called trace elements. The only difference in the collection is that the blood must be collected in a special tube that is metal-free. These are usually royal-blue-stoppered tubes that will or will not contain an anticoagulant.

Therapeutic Phlebotomy

Polycythemia is a disease that causes an increase in the number of erythrocytes in a patient's blood. One method of treating the disease is through the use of therapeutic phlebotomy. Therapeutic phlebotomy is done to draw large amounts of blood from the patient. This reduces the strain on the heart and other body systems. The amount of blood taken at one treatment is 500 milliliters. This is done in the same manner as if the patient were making a donation of blood to a blood bank. The blood is then discarded and not used for someone else.

MAKING A BLOOD SMEAR

Blood smears are needed when a microscopic examination of the blood is required. Blood smears may be prepared from venous blood or from capillary blood. The most common blood smear is used for the CBC differential test. Blood smears are also made, for example, for malaria tests and special hematology procedures. The blood is smeared on a glass slide to produce a smear known as a wedge or thin smear. A good smear has a feathered edge that is nearly square and shows rainbow sheen when reflecting light. The perfect slide consists of a smear that is exactly one cell thick in the feathered edge.

It takes considerable practice to make good slides consistently. Slide-making devices are available. These are too large to carry with you and are designed to work with automated differential reading instruments. Some of these devices make an actual wedge smear; others spin the slide to create a single layer of cells over the entire slide. The handmade wedge or thin slide is the most commonly made blood film.

For malaria, microfilariae, and trypanosomes identification, a second type of blood film is also used. Called a thick smear, this is not a smear at all but consists of a large drop of blood about the size of a dime (2 centimeters in diameter) placed in the center of the slide and allowed to dry (Fig. 6.1). This thick drop of blood is then checked for the malarial plasmodium or other blood parasites.

GLUCOSE TESTING

Glucose testing is preferable on a patient that is **NPO**. Such a patient will have had nothing to eat or drink since the previous night and is in a fasting condition. A high fasting glucose level (hyperglycemia) could be indicative of a diabetic patient.

Diabetes mellitus is a complicated disease that has other effects on an individual besides an increased blood glucose level. Persons with diabetes mellitus often develop other complications such as blindness, kidney failure, or circulatory problems that result in tissue

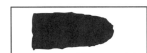
A. Bullet Smear

B. Straight Edge Smear

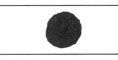
C. Malarial Thick Smear

fig 6.1 Blood smears

The class should practice making blood smears until each student can make consistent, good quality smears. The procedure for making a blood smear with a feathered edge is as follows and is shown in Fig. 6.2:

1. Select two glass slides that are clean and free of chipped edges. Fingerprints, grease, dust, or powder from gloves on the surface of the slides makes them unacceptable. Gloves should now be worn for the remaining steps of the procedure.

2. Place a drop of blood 1 to 2 millimeters in diameter on one of the slides. The drop should be in the center line approximately 1/4 inch from the frosted edge of the slide.

3. Hold the slide with the drop of blood at the opposite end with the thumb and forefinger of your nondominant hand. Grasp the spreader slide similarly with your dominant hand.

4. Rest the left end of the spreader slide at a 45° angle just in front of the drop of blood.

5. Draw the spreader slide backward until it just touches the drop of blood. Jiggle the spreader slide slightly to cause the the drop of blood to spread to the edges of the slide. The blood must spread evenly along the interface of the two slides. Not spreading the blood evenly causes a rounded feathered edge.

6. Keep the spreader slide at the 45° angle. Push the spreader slide rapidly across the stationary slide with even stroke and pressure. Any pressure exerted on the spreader slide should be directed across the slide in the direction that the film is made rather than down on the stationary slide. The slower the spreader slide is moved, the longer and thinner the film will be. The faster the slide is moved, the shorter and thicker the film will be. The angle will also vary the slide. An angle greater than 45° will make the smear thicker. An angle less than 45° will make the smear thinner. Speed, angle, and drop size can be varied slightly to produce a good smear.

7. Allow the slide to air dry. To facilitate air drying, fan the slide back and forth by holding between thumb and forefinger.

8. Check the slide for acceptability. The smear should cover approximately three-fourths of the length of the slide. The feathered edge should be either straight or bullet-shaped (Fig. 6.1). The preference of a straight or bullet smear is laboratory-directed. The edge should have a rainbow appearance when reflecting light. The smear should be smooth the entire length of the slide. There should be no holes or grainy appearance.

9. Write the patient information on the slide using pencil (ink from a ballpoint pen will wash off when the slide is processed). The patient information is written on the slide at the thick end of the smear.

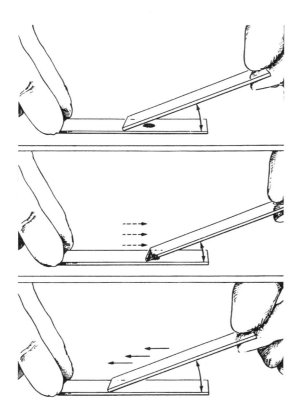

fig 6.2 Blood film preparation

damage and possible lower limb amputation. Hyperglycemia is the signal that a person may have diabetes mellitus. These patients often have fasting blood glucose levels within normal limits but are unable properly to metabolize ingested glucose. The glucose tolerance test (GTT) detects the borderline diabetic by measuring the ability to dispose of a large oral intake of glucose.

A fasting blood specimen is obtained, as well as a urine specimen. The glucose level of the blood and the presence or absence of glucose in the urine are then determined. Depending on the result of the glucose analysis, one of the following courses of action should be taken. In general, if the fasting glucose specimen is greater than 140 milligrams per deciliter, no GTT is necessary; if the fasting specimen is less than 140 milligrams per deciliter, then the GTT should be completed. Different laboratories use different values to determine whether a GTT is needed.

The patient is given a loading dose of glucose in the form of a flavored drink that contains a large amount of glucose. There is still some debate as to what constitutes an ideal loading dose of glucose. Some institutions give a set amount of glucose, either 75 grams or 100 grams of glucose, regardless of patient size. Other institutions base the amount of glucose on the patient's size. The dose is based on 40 grams of glucose per square meter of body surface. Charts that are available use the patient's height and weight to calculate the amount of glucose drink to give the person.

Blood specimens are then drawn at 30 minutes, 1 hour, 2 hours, 3 hours, and so on, after the dose. At each of these times, a urine specimen is also collected. The glucose tolerance test is carried out for the length of time the physician has requested. This is generally 3 to 5 hours. The values obtained through a glucose tolerance test can be graphed to

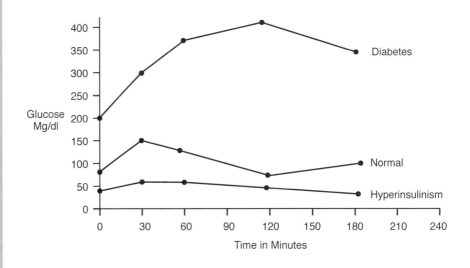

determine the severity of the diabetes compared to normal (Fig. 6.3). The same type of blood specimen must be obtained for the entire test. If venous blood is collected for the fasting specimen, all specimens collected must be venous blood. A capillary fasting specimen dictates that capillary blood be collected for the remainder of the test. Any specimens collected in tubes without a preservative must be centrifuged immediately to prevent glycolysis.

Postprandial Glucose Test

Instead of starting with a glucose tolerance test, the physician will often order a specimen be drawn for a blood sugar test 2 hours after a meal. A normal patient's blood glucose will not be elevated 2 hours after a meal. A diabetic patient will have an elevated glucose level after a meal. The **postprandial** glucose test is used as a screening test after a patient has shown elevated levels on a fasting blood glucose test.

Two-Hour Postglucose Drink

Giving a patient a glucose load as in a glucose tolerance test and then measuring the glucose level 2 hours later is more objective than the postprandial glucose test. This method

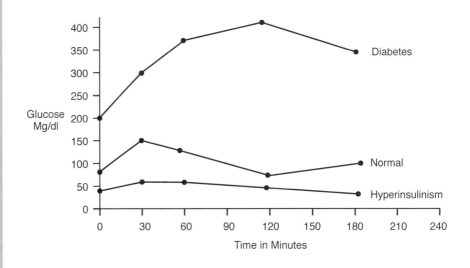

fig 6.3 Glucose tolerance test

EXERCISE 51 GLUCOSE TOLERANCE TEST

The instructor selects a time for a glucose tolerance test to be started and tolerance beverage given. Each student turns in to the instructor the times urine and blood would be collected for a 4-hour glucose tolerance test.

standardizes the amount of glucose given and eliminates the variables of time to consume the meal and time to absorb the meal. The patient has the benefit of not having blood drawn as many times as with a glucose tolerance test.

Home Monitoring of Glucose

Persons with diabetes do not want to go to a laboratory to be tested on a daily basis. Several instruments for home monitoring are available for patient purchase. All the instruments use the same basic principle. The patient performs a fingerstick and puts a drop of blood on a small testing pad. The pad is then inserted into the instrument, and at the proper time the glucose value is read. The patient records the value and can be trained to adjust the insulin dose depending on the glucose values.

BLEEDING TIMES

Bleeding time is the time it takes a standardized wound to stop bleeding. When a vessel is injured in a patient with normal coagulation function, platelets adhere to the exposed wound and lining of the vessel. Platelets then aggregate at the wound site, forming the primary platelet plug. Bleeding time is a measure of the functional integrity of the small blood vessels and the ability of platelets to form hemostatic plugs to stop bleeding. Bleeding time is prolonged in diseases that affect the ability of vessels to constrict and retract and in diseases in which the platelet number is decreased (thrombocytopenia). Diseases such as thrombasthenia and thrombocytopathy, which decrease platelet function, also cause an increase in bleeding time. Aspirin, aspirin-containing drugs, certain anticoagulants, antibiotics, and antihistamines prolong the bleeding time in normal patients. Any aspirin or other drugs that prolong bleeding time should be eliminated for one week before the test.

It is important to know that bleeding time is affected most when the platelet count falls below 100,000 per cubic millimeter. It is good practice to have a platelet count on the patient before bleeding time is determined. It is fruitless to expect a bleeding time to be normal when the platelet count is decreased.

Several different methods are available. Devices can be purchased that make one or two incisions. Figure 6.4 shows a single incision device called Surgicutt, produced by the International Technidyne Corporation of Edison, NJ. The Surgicutt device uses an automated incision-making device to make the cut for the bleeding time test. The device is spring-loaded and provides a standard cut 5 millimeters in length and 1 millimeter in depth. When triggered, the blade protracts down, sweeps across, and automatically retracts back into the device. This retraction of the blade is a safety feature to prevent accidental cutting of the phlebotomist with a contaminated lancet.

THE BLOOD CULTURE

Blood cultures are collected whenever it is suspected that a patient has **septicemia**. Septicemia is a condition in which microorganisms (mainly bacteria) circulate and multiply in a patient's blood. Since blood is normally sterile, the presence of microorganisms and their products is very serious and can result in death. The blood is collected and placed in a bottle that contains a solution that enhances the growth of significant microorganisms. An anticoagulant is also present. The microorganisms can then be cultured and identified so the most effective antibiotic treatment can be started.

EXERCISE 52 SURGICUTT BLEEDING TIME METHOD

Reagents and Equipment

Sphygmomanometer (blood pressure cuff)

Surgicutt bleeding time device

Circle filter paper (No. 11, Whatman, Inc., Clifton, NJ)

Stopwatch

Alcohol wipes

Gauze pads

Wound closure strip

Gloves

Procedure

1. Verify patient identity.

2. Apply gloves before any patient contact.

3. Place the patient's arm on a steady support with the volar surface exposed. The incision is best performed over the lateral aspect, volar surface of the forearm, parallel to and 5 centimeters below the antecubital crease. Avoid surface scars, bruises, surface veins, and edematous areas.

4. Place the sphygmomanometer cuff on the patient's upper arm. Inflate the cuff and maintain pressure at 40 millimeters of mercury The time between inflation of cuff and incision should be no more than 30 seconds. Hold at this exact pressure for the duration of the test (Fig. 6.4, step 1).

5. Clean the outer surface of the patient's forearm with alcohol; allow to air dry (Fig. 6.4, step 2).

6. Remove the Surgicutt device from the pack, being careful not to contaminate the instrument by touching or resting the blade-slot end on any unsterile surface (Fig. 6.4, step 3).

7. Remove the safety clip. Do not push the trigger or touch the blade slot (Fig. 6.4, step 4).

8. Observe the patient's forearm for superficial veins. Determine a location away from any superficial veins. Gently rest the device on the patient's forearm at the location selected and apply minimal pressure so that both ends of the device are lightly touching the skin. The incision is best performed parallel to the anticubital crease (Fig. 6.4, step 5).

9. Gently push the trigger and start the stopwatch simultaneously.

10. Remove the device from the patient's forearm immediately after triggering. (Fig. 6.4, step 6).

11. Blot the blood with filter paper at regular 30-second intervals. Do not touch the paper directly to the incision, so as not to disturb the platelet plug (Fig. 6.4, step 7).

12. Wick the blood every 30 seconds from then on until blood no longer stains the paper. Stop the timer. Bleeding time is determined to the nearest 30 seconds (Fig. 6.4, step 8).

13. Remove the sphygmomanometer cuff and cleanse the area with an alcohol swab. The potential for scarring and keloiding can be reduced by closing the edges of the incision with a wound closure strip for 24 hours (Fig. 6.4, step 9). Inform the patient that there will be a small scar present after healing.

Normals   2 to 8 minutes

Comments   If the patient continues to bleed after 15 minutes, stop the test and apply pressure to the wound.

Hints on Technique

1. The pressure placed on the Surgicutt device will affect the bleeding time.

2. The incision may be made either parallel or perpendicular to the anticubital crease. Results will vary depending on the direction of the incision; therefore, one direction should be used consistently.

3. Blood should flow freely within 20 seconds.

If blood cultures are to be collected after antimicrobial treatment has started, the blood culture must be drawn in a special bottle containing a resin solution to inactivate the antimicrobial agent. This will then allow the bacteria to grow. The resin bottle is known as an Antibiotic Removal Device (ARD) bottle.

The volume of blood needed is critical to optimum recovery of the microorganisms. Up to 10 milliliters of blood are to be placed in the bottle. The optimum amount of blood varies depending on the manufacturer of the blood culture bottles. For infants and children, 1 to 5 milliliters of blood in a pediatric bottle is sufficient.

The blood cultures are drawn in sets of two bottles. One bottle is a aerobic bottle for those microorganisms that need oxygen to grow. The second bottle is an anaerobic bottle for microorganisms requiring an environment without oxygen. A set of blood cultures used to be collected at the height of the patient's fever. This is when the microorganisms were thought to be at their greatest number in the blood. With the new high-recovery blood culture bottles available, drawing of blood at the height of fever is not as critical. Even during a low point of fever, the microorganisms are present in sufficient number for rapid growth. Two blood culture sets are sufficient for recovery of significant microorganisms. Ideally, the two sets are taken at separate venipuncture sites before therapy is started.

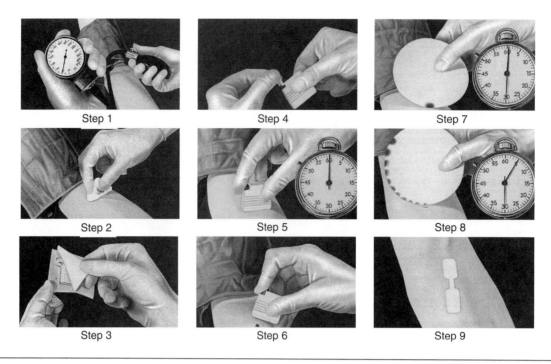

Step 1 Step 4 Step 7
Step 2 Step 5 Step 8
Step 3 Step 6 Step 9

fig 6.4 Surgicutt bleeding time procedure

The most critical step in collecting a blood culture is proper cleaning of the site. The site must be as clean as possible to avoid contaminating the blood culture with skin-surface microorganisms, thus producing a false-positive blood culture. As with most techniques, the cleaning procedure varies from one laboratory to another.

After the site is cleaned, the seals on the bottles are broken off. This seal usually consists of a metal flip-off cap. Under the seal is a rubber septum through which the blood is injected. Once the flip-off cap is removed, the septum is cleaned with an alcohol pad. Iodine should not be used. The alcohol pad is left on the bottle until just before the blood is injected. The proper amount of blood is then drawn with a syringe.

Instead of using a syringe to draw the blood and inoculate the bottles, a butterfly collection set can be used (Refer to Unit 4). The Becton Dickinson company produces a BACTEC Direct Draw Adapter that attaches to the rubber-sleeved end of the butterfly, as is normally done with the vacutainer holder (Fig. 6.5). The top of each bottle is cleaned with alcohol. The patient's vein is accessed with the butterfly needle. The Direct Draw Adapter is then slipped over the top of the anaerobic bottle and then the aerobic bottle. Once the needle punctures the bottle, the bottle will begin to fill with blood. Each bottle is filled to the proper level of blood. Once the blood cultures are collected, additional tubes of blood can be drawn without "sticking" the patient again.

Other blood culture bottles have a long neck that will insert into an evacuated needle holder. The tops of the bottles are cleaned with alcohol. The blood is drawn directly into the special bottle, and the media is directly inoculated. The blood culture media can be indirectly inoculated by using the Isolator collection tube manufactured by Wampole. The microbiology laboratory uses this tube to inoculate directly on solid culture media to determine if microorganisms are present.

All blood culture methods call for some variation in procedure for the phlebotomist. The arm-cleaning technique has variations in procedure. Some blood culture systems must

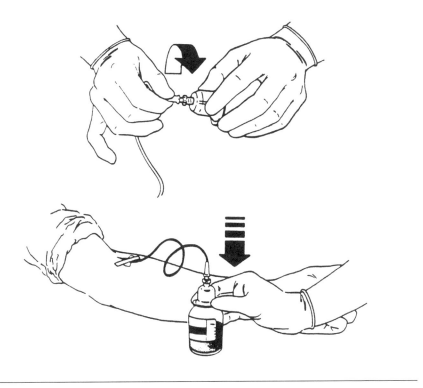

fig 6.5 BACTEC Direct Draw Adapter (*courtesy of Becton Dickinson BACTEC Systems*)

E X E R C I S E   53   CLEANING A BLOOD CULTURE COLLECTION SITE

Each student cleans the back of her or his own hand as if they are going to do a blood culture venipuncture.

1. Clean the site with alcohol to remove the oils and dirt on the skin surface.

2. The site is then cleaned with a 2 percent tincture of iodine solution.

3. The cleaning is done with a circular motion, starting at the site of the puncture and moving in concentric circles outward.

4. The iodine is painted on the area, not flooded over the site. Iodine is an effective antiseptic only if it is allowed to dry before the venipuncture is attempted.

Caution: Before any cleaning of the site is begun, the patient must be asked if he or she is allergic to iodine. If the patient does have an iodine allergy, the only recourse is to clean thoroughly with 70 percent alcohol.

EXERCISE 54 BLOOD CULTURE COLLECTION

Using an anatomical arm, collect one set of blood cultures.

1. Remove protective sealer from the top of each blood culture bottle.

2. Clean the top of each bottle with an alcohol swab. Leave swab on top of bottle until after the blood has been drawn.

3. Select the vein before cleaning the site.

4. Clean the site as was done in Exercise 53.

5. Using a syringe, draw 15 milliliters of blood.

6. Remove the alcohol pad from the bottle top.

7. Without changing needles, inject the appropriate amount of blood into the bottles. Always inject the anaerobic bottle first to maintain a strict anaerobic environment.

8. Label all bottles before leaving the patient's bedside.

have the aerobic bottle vented (air added) by the phlebotomist. A variation in procedure does not indicate the laboratory is improper but illustrates variations in manufacturers.

FACTORS AFFECTING LABORATORY VALUES

Numerous variables can affect test results. Once some of these variables come into play, the most expensive analytical instrument on the market cannot give an accurate and precise result. Some of these factors are the responsibility of the phlebotomist; others reflect the physiological factors of the patient (Table 6.1).

Certain specimens require immediate chilling after collection (Table 6.2). This is done by placing the specimen into ice as you withdraw it from the evacuated tube holder. Any delay in icing the specimen will alter test results. The longer the delay, the greater the change.

The phlebotomist is not the only person who may affect test results. The patient can knowingly or unknowingly alter the results by certain actions. Patients will often say they have had nothing to eat or drink and will have had a cup of coffee. The patient is often under the misconception that black coffee without sugar will not be a problem. Coffee and smoking affect the metabolism and can affect test results.

URINE, SEMEN, AND THROAT CULTURE COLLECTION

Urine Collection

Urine is the most common specimen that the patient collects himself or herself. The laboratory should provide the collection container to assure the cleanliness of the container used. For specimens that will be used for culture, the container must be sterile. All specimens, with the exception of 24-hour collections, are best collected as clean-catch mid-stream urine. At times the specimen will need to be collected with a catheter by a qualified associate. Patient cooperation is needed for any urine specimen to be accurate. The urine specimens can vary depending on the timing of collection, as shown in Table 6.3.

Table **6–1**   Factors Affecting Results

Factor	Effect on Test Result
Tourniquet	Hemoconcentration, change in analyte concentration
Fasting	Patient not in fasting state; results of tests will not be accurate
Diurnal rhythm	Some specimens must be drawn at timed intervals because of medication or diurnal rhythm. The exact time of collection must also be noted on the specimen.
Heparin	Incorrect heparin used; result affected
Exercise	Strenuous short-term exercise can make the heart work harder and increase the heart enzymes. Long-term exercise such as undergone by highly trained runners, can lead to runner's anemia.
Stress	Stress can have an effect similer to exercise. In children, violent crying before a specimen is collected will raise the WBC count up to 146 percent.
Volume	Not enough blood will cause a dilutional factor, changing the size of the cells or causing variation in test results.

E X E R C I S E **55**   **TUBE QUALITY CONTROL**

Defective tubes give an improper fill even with the best venipuncture. Tubes should vary no more than $+/-10$ percent in filling. A syringe filled with water should be used to determine the quality of the tubes.

1. Each student takes a syringe with needle attached and fills it with water.

2. The syringe should be filled with more water than the capacity of tube that is being tested.

3. The student then takes five evacuated tubes.

4. The top of the tube is punctured with the syringe needle, and the amount of water the tube pulls from the syringe is noted.

5. The number of tubes that vary more than 10 percent from the stated volume are counted for the class.

6. The class then calculates the percentage of tubes that are defective.

Table 6-2 Examples of Common Tests Requiring Chilling of the Specimen

1. Ammonia
2. Catecholamines
3. Gastrin
4. Lactic acid
5. Parathyroid hormone (PTH)
6. pH/blood gas

Table 6-3 Types of Urine Collections

Random	Collected at any time.
First morning	Collected when the patient first arises from a night's sleep.
8-hour	Collected after 8 hours' sleep, usually used for night workers who sleep during the day.
Double-voided	The patient collects a urine sample and then drinks 200 milliliters of water. The urine is allowed to accumulate in the bladder for a specified time, and then a second specimen is collected.
Timed	Specimen is collected at a specific time during a 24-hour period. An example is 2 hours after a meal. Blood may also be obtained at the same time.
24-hour	The patient voids and discards the first morning specimen. All urine, including the next morning specimen, is then saved. The patient must cooperate and not discard a single specimen.

When urine testing is delayed for more than 1 hour after the specimen is collected, special precautions must be taken. This is necessary to avoid both deterioration of chemical and cellular elements in the urine, and the multiplication of microorganisms. Multiplication of microorganisms causes a decrease in the urine glucose level. Microorganisms also cause a change in pH, affecting all cellular elements present. Refrigeration at 5° Celsius is often the only way to preserve the urine for routine analysis. Chemical preservatives are used as an alternative in most 24-hour urine specimens and in urine that cannot be refrigerated.

Semen Collection

Semen specimens are used to determine the number and activity of sperm contained in the semen. This can be done as a part of a fertility study and also postvasectomy to determine if the vasectomy was successful.

Masturbation into a sterile container is the preferred method of collection. Condoms often contain lubricants and powders that are injurious to sperm; they should not be used for collection. After the specimen is obtained, it is important to deliver it to the laboratory within 1 hour and to protect it from any extremes of temperature. Placing the container in a shirt or pants pocket will generally assure that the temperature will remain proper. The laboratory must know the exact time of collection.

A phlebotomist working in a clinic or outpatient setting will be involved in the collection of various types of cultures, including cultures of the throat. A physician will order a culture for a patient with a sore throat. A swab is used to collect the specimen for culture. Commercial collection sets that contain swabs and transport (holding) media are the collection methods of choice.

E X E R C I S E 56 URINE COLLECTION

The class divides into four groups. After discussion a representative of each group presents to the class:

1. what a patient might do to invalidate a 24-hour urine collection
2. how a patient could collect all the urine during a 24-hour period and still go to work
3. how the group would keep a urine specimen cold when the patient had to work

E X E R C I S E 57 COLLECTING A THROAT CULTURE

The procedure for proper throat culture collection is demonstrated to the class by the instructor on a volunteer student. The students divide into pairs, and each pair performs a throat culture on one student.

1. Collect equipment needed, including sterile swab, tongue depressor, and gloves.
2. Position patient so that the head is tilted back.
3. Depress the patient's tongue with the tongue depressor, and ask the patient to say "ah."
4. Be careful not to touch the swab to the mouth or tongue surface, because these surfaces have microorganisms that can interfere with the growth of potential pathogens.
5. Swab the back of the throat and surfaces of the tonsils with the sterile swab. Be gentle; this area is often inflamed and painful.

SPECIMEN PRESERVATION AND TRANSPORT

Specimens, once collected, must be transported. Any transportation within the facility is usually done by the phlebotomist or a transporter. When a specimen is transported, the primary container in which the specimen was collected must be placed in a secondary container so that any leakage or breakage of the primary container is contained. A sealable plastic bag is sufficient as the secondary container for most specimens. A single specimen can be placed in the bag, and then the bag can be sealed shut. Large numbers of specimens can be placed in racks to avoid spillage or breakage, and the entire rack can be placed in a leakproof box. Standard camping coolers, which come in various sizes, are excellent for this purpose. Whatever secondary container is used, the biohazard emblem must be attached.

Some institutions have pneumatic tube systems or robots to transport specimens. This type of transport can be more traumatic to the specimen than hand carrying but has the advantage of faster delivery. Transporting specimens over long distances requires more precautions to avoid leakage of the specimen outside the packaging.

The integrity of a specimen must be maintained during shipment. Extreme variation in temperature must be avoided during both long- and short-distance transport. The maximum time the specimen will take to arrive at the destination must be determined, and then the appropriate amount of dry ice or insulation must be added to protect the specimen.

SUMMARY

The phlebotomist will often be required to have a knowledge of special specimen requirements for certain procedures. The procedures can require that the phlebotomist confirm whether the patient has had anything to eat or drink, or when was the last time the patient had a meal. Therapeutic drug monitoring requires the phlebotomist to check before a venipuncture is made to verify that a drug has not been given and then to check again to be certain all the drug was given.

The phlebotomist will have to prioritize the draws when STAT procedures are ordered. The phlebotomist will often have to change the order of patients to draw a STAT specimen and have it processed as rapidly as possible. Blood cultures require a special cleaning procedure for the venipuncture site to prevent contamination of the sample. Many other factors in transportation and handling of the specimen can affect laboratory results.

The role of the phlebotomist is not always restricted to blood. The phlebotomist in some health care positions is required to give patients instructions in urine and semen collection.

REVIEW QUESTIONS

Choose the one best answer.

1 The glucose tolerance test is used to help in the diagnosis of:
a. heart problems
b. diabetes
c. liver function
d. cancer

2 Which of the following statements concerning bleeding time measurement is true?
a. You must touch only the drop of blood, not the skin, with the filter paper.
b. A stop watch must be started at the same time that the puncture is made.
c. The test is done to assess platelet function.
d. All of the above are true.

3 In which test must alcohol never be used to cleanse the venipuncture site?
a. Blood cultures
b. HIV test
c. Alcohol test
d. Platelet count

4 Which of the following is the antiseptic(s) of choice for blood culture collection?
a. 0.5 percent chlorhexidine gluconate
b. 70 percent isopropyl alcohol
c. 1 to 2 percent tincture of iodine
d. both 1 to 2 percent tincture of iodine and 70 percent isopropyl alcohol

5 What is the best specimen for urine culture?
a. Any random specimen
b. A catheterized specimen
c. A clean-catch midstream urine specimen
d. A specimen from an "ostomy" bag

FURTHER ACTIVITIES

The throat sample taken in Exercise 57 is inoculated on agar medium and incubated. The bacterial growth is shown to the class during the next class period.

The instructor plots glucose tolerance values for the class and illustrates different diabetic risks.

The instructor demonstrates different types of blood culture bottles and the variations in sample collection for each type of bottle.

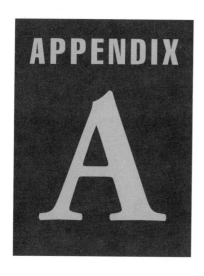

Sources of Phlebotomist Certification

- PBT(ASCP): Phlebotomy Technician.
  American Society of Clinical Pathologists
- RPT(AMT): Registered Phlebotomy Technician,
  American Medical Technologists
- CPT(ASPT): Certified Phlebotomy Technician,
  American Society of Phlebotomy Technicians
- CPT(IAPSI): Certified Phlebotomy Technician,
  International Academy of Phlebotomy Sciences, Inc.
- CLP(NCA): Clinical Laboratory Phlebotomist,
  National Certification Agency for Medical Laboratory Personnel
- CPT(NPA): Phlebotomy Technician,
  National Phlebotomy Association

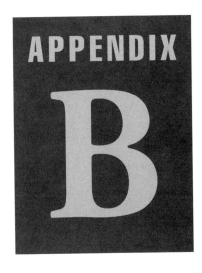

Patient Rights

In support of increased ethical treatment of patients and patient relation awareness, the American Hospital Association in 1973 drafted and approved a Patient's Bill of Rights. Their goals in implementing this are to contribute to more effective care. The Patient's Bill of Rights will ensure greater satisfaction of the patient, physician, and hospital. Support of these rights by a hospital will become an integral part of the healing process. This Bill of Rights existed before the onset of AIDS and before many new medical procedures, but it still is very up-to-date in its substance. By examining the Bill of Rights, we will be able to see how, by following these rights, we can ensure that the patient will be treated ethically and professionally.

PATIENT'S BILL OF RIGHTS

"The American Hospital Association presents a Patient's Bill of Rights with the expectation that observance of these rights will contribute to more effective patient care and greater satisfaction for the patient, his physician, and the hospital organization. Further, the Association presents these rights in the expectation that they will be supported by the hospital on behalf of its patients, and an integral part of the healing process. It is recognized that a personal relationship between the physician and the patient is essential for the provision of proper medical care. The traditional physician–patient relationship takes on a new dimension when care is rendered within an organizational structure. Legal precedent has established that the institution itself also has a responsibility to the patient. It is in recognition of these factors that these rights are affirmed.

1 The patient has the right to considerate and respectful care.

2 The patient has the right to obtain from his physician complete current information concerning his diagnosis, treatment, and prognosis in terms the patient can be reasonably expected to understand. When it is not medically advisable to give such information to the patient, the information should be made available to an appropriate person in his behalf. He has the right to know, by name, the physician responsible for coordinating his care.

3 The patient has the right to receive from his physician information necessary to

give informed consent prior to the start of any procedure and/or treatment. Except in emergencies, such information for informed consent should include but not necessarily be limited to the specific procedure and/or treatment, the medically significant risks involved, and the probable duration of incapacitation. Where medically significant alternatives for care or treatment exist, or when the patient requests information concerning medical alternatives, the patient has the right to such information. The patient has the right to know the name of the person responsible for the procedures and/or treatment.

4 The patient has the right to refuse treatment to the extent permitted by law and to be informed of the medical consequences of his actions.

5 The patient has the right to every consideration of his privacy concerning his own medical care program. Case discussion, consultation, examination, and treatment are confidential and should be considered discreetly. Those not directly involved in his care must have the permission of the patient to be present.

6 The patient has the right to expect that all communications and records pertaining to his care should be treated as confidential.

7 The patient has the right to expect that within its capacity a hospital must make reasonable response to the request of a patient for services. The hospital must provide evaluation, service, and/or referral as indicated by the urgency of the case. When medically permissible, a patient may be transferred to another facility only after he has received complete information and explanation concerning the needs for and alternatives to such a transfer. The institution to which the patient is to be transferred must have accepted the patient for transfer.

8 The patient has the right to obtain information as to any relationship of his hospital to other health care and educational institutions to the extent that his care is concerned. The patient has the right to obtain information as to the existence of any professional relationships among individuals, by name, who are treating him.

9 The patient has the right to be advised if the hospital proposes to engage in or perform human experimentation affecting his care or treatment. The patient has the right to refuse to participate in such projects.

10 The patient has the right to expect reasonable continuity of care. He has the right to know in advance what appointment times and physicians are available and where. The patient has the right to expect that the hospital will provide a mechanism whereby he is informed by his physician or a delegate of the physician of the patient's continuing health care requirements following discharge.

11 The patient has the right to examine and receive an explanation of his bill regardless of source of payment.

12 The patient has the right to know what hospital rules and regulations apply to his conduct as a patient.

No catalog of rights can guarantee for the patient the kind of treatment he has the right to expect. A hospital has many functions to perform, including the prevention and treatment of disease, the education of both health professionals and patients, and the conduct of clinical research. All these activities must be conducted with an overriding concern for the patient, and, above all, the recognition of his dignity as a human being. Success in achieving this recognition assures success in the defense of the rights of the patient."

Most of these rights can be directly related to the duties of a phlebotomist.

1 The patient has the right to considerate and respectful care. Hospitalized patients are out of their normal routine. They may react by being rude or ill-tempered, due to their illness or fear. Some patients may be confronting the realization of their own mortality for the first time. It is important for the phlebotomist to remain calm and to show consideration and concern for each patient. The phlebotomist must face the realization of mortality. In the United States, 85 percent of the population will die in hospital. The phlebotomist will at some time walk into a patient's room and find the patient deceased. Sometimes this will be even before anyone else has been aware of the death. Even in times of death, the patient must be treated with respect.

2 The physician is the patient's primary source concerning diagnosis and treatment. If questions are asked during the phlebotomy procedure, simply state that the doctor has ordered blood to be drawn for testing and refer the patient to the physician. The phlebotomist may question the need for the test to be drawn or realize that an error with a previous specimen necessitates redrawing the patient's blood. Questions and concerns should not be discussed with the patient but with the phlebotomist's supervisor or the nurse, outside the presence of the patient.

3 Informed consent: The phlebotomist may need to briefly explain how the venipuncture is to be performed and that these are tests that the doctor has ordered. The patient's act of extending an arm for the procedure is taken as an act of consent.

4 Right to refuse treatment: Often by just talking with a patient, the phlebotomist can persuade the patient to consent to the procedure. If the patient still refuses, the nursing staff and physician must be informed.

5 Consideration of privacy: It is important to remember to be discreet in approaching to the patient. Often, the phlebotomist is in the room at the time another procedure is being performed, the patient is completing personal hygiene, or the physician is examining the patient. Under all of these circumstances, it is necessary to approach the situation in a mature fashion.

6 Confidentiality: Knowledge concerning a patient's diagnosis is confidential. Matters pertaining to a patient's care should not be discussed in the cafeteria, hallways, or other public areas. With such information, use discretion. Confidentiality can be broken as innocently, for example, as when the phlebotomist finds out that a friend of the family is pregnant and goes home to tell his/her spouse. The spouse then tells someone else, and all the relatives know before the pregnant relative has had the opportunity to tell anyone.

7 The patient has the right to expect a reasonable response to requests for services. The appropriate person to handle these requests is the nurse and/or physician. Often, a patient may request, for example, a drink of water, or aid in getting out of bed from a phlebotomist. Refer these requests to the nursing staff because the physician may have written specific orders denying the privilege due to upcoming surgery or other aspects related to that patient's care.

8 The patient has the right to know of professional relationships and the names of those who are rendering care. A patient may request to know the phlebotomist's name and title, and it is appropriate for you to give this information.

9 Experimentation: Patients who are involved in a medical experiment, be it a new drug or treatment, must first be informed of the proposed course of action. The patient must also be informed of its ramifications and must give informed consent to participate in the study.

10 Continuity of care: In these days of multiple specialties and treatment by several physicians at once, it is important to maintain continuity in the care and treatment of patients. For the laboratory, this means that specimens should be obtained and processed expeditiously to facilitate the care of the patient.

11 The patient has the right to examine and receive an explanation of his or her bill. Every care should be taken to ensure that the patient is charged for only those tests that are performed and that billing is handled expeditiously.

12 The patient has the right to know the hospital rules and regulations that pertain to his or her conduct as a patient.

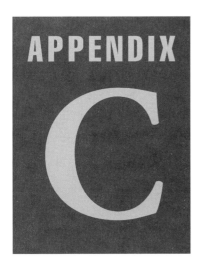

APPENDIX C

Answers to Review Questions

UNIT 1

1. D
2. D
3. B
4. C
5. D
6. D

UNIT 2

1. B
2. C
3. A
4. D
5. C
6. D
7. B

UNIT 3

1. C
2. D
3. F
4. D
5. C

UNIT 4

1 B
2 A
3 D
4 C
5 B
6 C
7 C
8 B
9 B
10 B
11 C
12 A

UNIT 5

1 C
2 C
3 A
4 A
5 D
6 B
7 B
8 C
9 C
10 D

UNIT 6

1 B
2 D
3 C
4 D
5 C

REFERENCES

Bissell, Michael, and Teri Cosman. "How Ethical Dilemmas Induce Stress," *Medical Laboratory Observer.* July 1991, pp. 28–33.

Blumenfeld, TA, GK Turi, and WA Blanc. "Recommended Site and Depth of Newborn Heel Skin Punctures Based on Anatomical Measurements and Histopathology," *Lancet.* 1979;1:230–233.

Daigneault, MT(ASCP)SH, Robert. "A Surprise Visit from OSHA," *Medical Laboratory Observer.* January 1990, pp. 31–34.

Doyle, Edward T. "Protecting Laboratory Workers," *MT Today.* December 16, 1991, pp. 1–9.

Federal Register, Rules and Regulations, 29 CFR Part 1910.1030. Vol. 56, (235), December 6, 1991.

Garner, JS, and BP Simmons. *CDC Guideline for Isolation Precautions in Hospitals.* Springfield, Virginia: National Technical Information Service, 1983.

Geller, Shayna J. *Effect of Sample Collection on Laboratory Test Results.* ASCP Teleconference Series, March 3, 1992.

Gylys, Barbara A, and Mary Ellen Wedding. *Medical Terminology: A Systems Approach.* Philadelphia: F. A. Davis Company, 1988, pp. 145–156.

Hay, Karen. "The Making of a Blood Film." *Designs for Learning.* Kettering Medical Center, 1979.

Hoeltke, Lynn B. "How Internships Eased our Phlebotomist Shortage," *Medical Laboratory Observer.* May 1991, pp. 65–72.

Hoeltke, Lynn B. *The Complete Textbook of Phlebotomy.* Albany, N.Y.: Delmar Publishers, 1994.

Mobley, MHE MT (ASCP), C. Regina, and Vern Simon, MA MT (ASCP). "Coping With CLIA," *Diagnostics.* Vol. 27, 9:18–20, November/December 1989.

Moya, M.D., Carlos E, Luis A Guarda, M.D., and Thomas M Sodeman, M.D. "Safety in the Clinical Laboratory. Part 1: Hazard Identification System; and Part 2: Fire Protection, Prevention and Control." *Laboratory Medicine.* Vol. 11, No. 9, September 1980, pp. 576–581.

National Committee for Clinical Laboratory Standards. *Blood Alcohol Testing in the Clinical Laboratory,* 2nd. ed. Approved Standard. NCCLS document T/DM6–P. Villanova, Pennsylvania 19085, 1988.

National Committee for Clinical Laboratory Standards. *Blood Collection on Filter Paper for Neonatal Screening Programs,* 2nd. ed. Approved Standard. NCCLS document LA4–A2. Villanova, Pennsylvania 19085, July 1992.

National Committee for Clinical Laboratory Standards. *Devices for Collection of Skin*

Puncture Blood Specimens, 2nd. ed. Approved Standard. NCCLS Document. H14–A2. Villanova, Pennsylvania 19085, 1990.

National Committee for Clinical Laboratory Standards. *Evacuated Tubes for Blood Specimen Collection.* Approved Standard. NCCLS Document. H1–A3. Villanova, Pennsylvania 19085, 1991.

National Committee for Clinical Laboratory Standards. *Percutaneous Collection of Arterial Blood for Laboratory Analysis.* Approved Standard. NCCLS document H11–A, Villanova, Pennsylvania 19085, 1985.

National Committee for Clinical Laboratory Standards. *Procedures for the Collection of Diagnostic Blood Specimens by Skin Puncture.* 3rd. ed. Approved Standard. NCCLS document H4–A3. Villanova, Pennsylvania 19085, 1991.

National Committee for Clinical Laboratory Standards. *Procedures for the Collection of Diagnostic Blood Specimens by Venipuncture,* 3rd. ed. Approved Standard. NCCLS document H3–A3. Villanova, Pennsylvania 19085, 1991.

National Committee for Clinical Laboratory Standards. *Procedures for the Domestic Handling and Transport of Diagnostic Specimens and Etiologic Agents,* 2nd ed. Approved Standard. NCCLS document H5–A2. Villanova, Pennsylvania 19085, 1985.

National Committee for Clinical Laboratory Standards. *Protection of Laboratory Workers from Infectious Disease Transmitted by Blood, Body Fluids, and Tissue,* 2nd. ed. Approved Standard. NCCLS Document. M29-T2, Villanova, Pennsylvania 19085, 1991.

Patient's Bill of Rights, *Hospitals.* Vol. 47, February 1973, p. 41.

Peek, GJ, H Marsh, J Keating, et al. "The Effects of Swabbing the Skin on Apparent Blood Ethanol Concentration." *Alcohol and Alcoholism.* 1990; 25:639–640.

Pittiglo, D Harmeniong, PhD, MT(ASCP), Ronald A. Sacher, MD, FRCP (C). *Clinical Hematology and Fundamentals of Hemostasis.* Philadelphia: F.A. Davis Company, 1987.

Procedures for Examination and Certification, Board of Registry. American Society of Clinical Pathologists, 1990.

Renner, B Charles, Samuel Meites, and John R Hayes. "Optimal Sites and Depths for Skin Puncture of Infants and Children as Assessed from Anatomical Measurements." *Clinical Chemistry* 1990;3:547–549.

Sisk, PhD, MT (ASCP), A Faye. "Trends in Regulation and Reimbursement," *Medical Laboratory Observer.* July 1991, pp. 49–55.

Slockbower, Jean M, and Thomas A Blumenfeld. *Collection and Handling of Laboratory Specimens.* Philadelphia: J.B. Lippincott Company, 1983.

Snyder, John R, Donald A Senhauser. *Administration and Supervision in Laboratory Medicine.* Philadelphia: J. B. Lippincott Company, 1989, pp. 33–38.

"Standardization of the Oral Glucose Tolerance Test: Report of the Committee on Statistics of the American Diabetes Association," *Diabetes.* 1969, 18: 299.

Surgicutt Package Insert. International Technidyne Corporation. Edison, N.J., 1992.

Technical Methods and Procedures of the American Association of Blood Banks, 10th ed. Philadelphia: J.B. Lippincott Company, 1990.

Tilton, Richard C, Albert Balows, David C Hohnadel, Robert F Reiss. *Clinical Laboratory Medicine.* St. Louis: Mosby–Year Book, Inc., 1992, pp. 813–823.

Trotto, Nancy E. "Certification of Laboratorians: An Update, "*Medical Laboratory Observer.* October 1991, pp. 26–36.

Wedding, Mary Ellen, Sally A Toenjes. *Medical Laboratory Procedures.* Philadelphia: F. A. Davis Company, 1992, pp. 3–5.

Page numbers in italic indicate figures.